RENAL DIET COOKBOOK

_____

_____

300 LOW SODIUM, POTASSIUM, AND PHOSPHORUS RECIPES WITH A 31-DAY MEAL PLAN INCLUDED. MANAGE KIDNEY DISEASE (CKD) & AVOID DIALYSIS

_____

_____

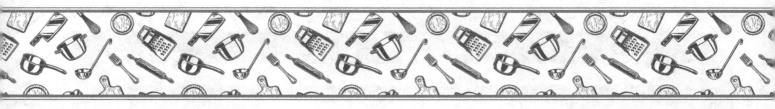

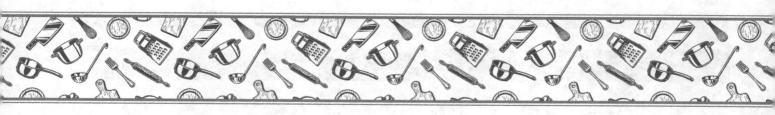

TABLE OF CONTENTS

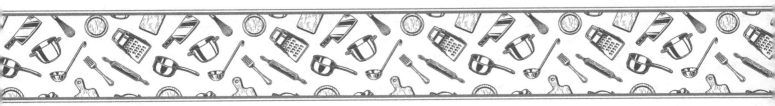

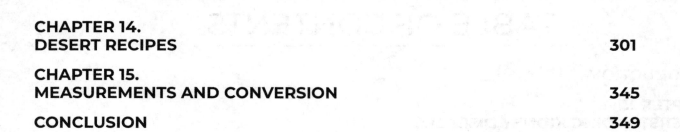

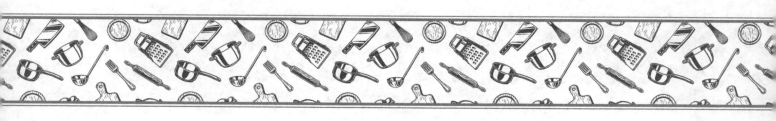

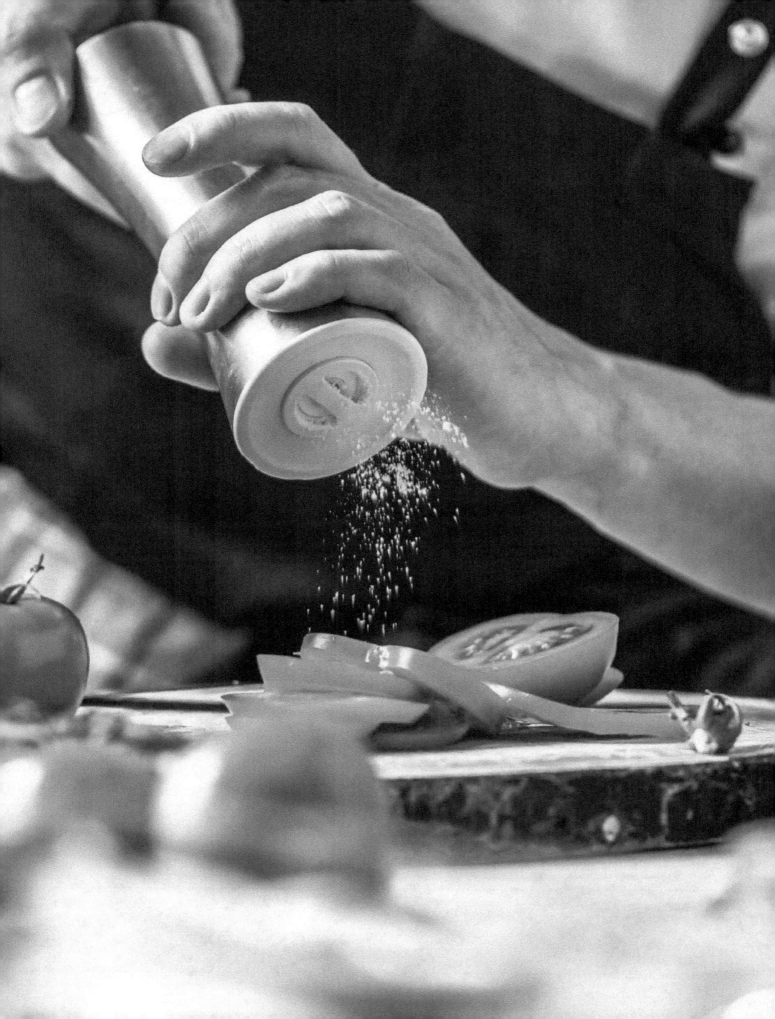

INTRODUCTION

Bad eating habits can have a lot of adverse effects on your health. If you want to avoid kidney diseases, you must manage a balanced diet and stay healthy. Your diet is supposed to contain low levels of fat and salt to control blood pressure. A diabetic person must maintain his/her blood sugar by choosing the right food and beverages to prevent the worse condition of kidney disease. Only a kidney-friendly diet can help you in the protection of kidneys from more damage. By choosing a kidney-friendly diet, you can limit particular foods to avoid the build-up of minerals in your body.

Salt or sodium is one of the essential ingredients that the renal diet prohibits its use. This ingredient, although simple, can badly and powerfully affect your body and especially the kidneys. Any excess of sodium can't be easily filtered because of the failing condition of the kidneys. A massive build-up of sodium can cause catastrophic results on your body. Potassium and Phosphorus are also prohibited for kidney patients depending on the stage of kidney disease.

Kidney disease or "renal disease" and "kidney damage" is a health condition where the kidneys cannot function healthily and properly. Chronic kidney disease is a slow-moving disease and does not cause the patient many complaints in the initial stages. Chronic kidney disease includes a group of kidney diseases, in which case the renal function decreases for several years or decades. With the help of timely diagnosis and treatment, it can slow down and even stop kidney disease progression.

Anatomically, the kidneys are positioned in the abdomen, at the back, usually on both sides of the spine. The renal artery, which is a direct branch of the aorta, supplies blood to the kidneys. Renal veins empty the blood from kidneys to the vena cava, then the heart. The word "renal" originated from the Latin word for kidney.

There is a special connection between the health and function of our kidneys and the way we eat. How we eat and the foods we choose make a significant impact on how well we feel and our overall well-being. Making changes to your diet is often necessary to guard against medical conditions. While eating well can treat existing conditions, healthy food choices can also help prevent many other conditions from developing – including kidney disease.

When we make changes to our diet, we often focus on the restrictions or foods we should avoid. While this is important, it's vital to learn about the foods and nutrients we need to maintain good health and prevent disease. Consider the related conditions that contribute to high blood pressure and type 2 diabetes. The dietary changes are often suggested to treat and, in some successful cases, reverse the damage of these conditions. Dietary changes for the treatment and prevention of disease often focus on limiting salt, sugar, and trans fats from our food choices, while increasing minerals, protein, and fiber, among other beneficial nutrients. The renal diet also focuses on eliminating, or at least limiting, the consumption of various ingredients to aid our kidneys to function better and to prevent further damage from occurring.

CHAPTER 1.
UNDERSTANDING KIDNEY DISEASES

Kidney function or renal functions are the terms used to explain how well the kidneys function. A healthy individual is born with a pair of kidneys. This is why whenever one of the kidneys lost its function, it went unnoticed due to the other kidney's function. But if the kidney functions further drop altogether and reach a level as low as 25 percent, it turns out to be serious for the patients. People who only have one functioning kidney need proper external therapy and, in worst cases, a kidney transplant.

Kidney diseases occur when a number of renal cells known as nephrons are either partially or completely damaged and fail to properly filter blood entering in. The gradual damage of the kidney cells can occur due to various reasons, sometimes it is the acidic or toxic build-up inside the kidney over time, at times it is genetic, or the result of other kidney damaging diseases like hypertension (high blood pressure) or diabetes.

Chronic Kidney Disease (CKD)

CKD or chronic kidney disease is the stage of kidney damage where it fails to filter the blood properly. The term chronic is used to refer to gradual and long-term damage to an organ. Chronic kidney disease is therefore developed after a slow yet progressive damage to the kidneys. The symptoms of this disease only appear when the toxic wastes start to build up in the body. Therefore, such a stage should be prevented at all costs. Hence, early diagnosis of the disease proves to be significant. The sooner the patient realizes the gravity of the situation, the better measures he can take to curb the problem.

What about after we are affected by diseases? Well, even then, we make sure that we spend less time pondering about and trying to change what we cannot and more time on how to take care of ourselves. By focusing on our own actions, we gain more confidence, motivation, and knowledge. We realize that the ability to make changes, however big or small, lies within us.

In the case of chronic kidney diseases, we have the power to ensure that the disease does not get worse.

Causes of Kidney Disease

According to the National Kidney Foundation, the two main causes of chronic kidney disease are high blood pressure and diabetes (National Kidney Foundation, n.d.). If you visit a doctor, health expert, or diet consultant, then you will realize that one of the major ways of managing your blood pressure and prevent diabetes is a healthy diet.

As the blood pressure or diabetes levels get worse, so does the amount of waste buildup. The waste goes into your blood faster than the kidneys are able to filter them. At this point, your kidneys are like an overworked employee at a firm; there is so much work still remaining but only a small amount of time to get finished during a particular period. The kidneys begin to deteriorate over time. The filters begin to leak, unable to hold on to the waste buildup anymore. Only a small percentage of the entire waste gets filtered properly, with the rest entering the bloodstream. For some, the time it takes for kidney failure might be months while for others, the kidneys could worsen across a span of years. It all depends on numerous factors like diet, lifestyle choices, and even genetics.

Pretty soon, you might feel like your kidney functions have been kidnapped; they don't seem to be functioning well anymore or they barely exist. But that is not the case. Think of the example of the overworked employee that we used earlier. At some point, the employee could collapse out of dehydration or exhaustion. In a similar way, kidney disease causes the organs to fail, which causes numerous problems such as low energy, high exhaustion levels, sleep difficulties, poor appetite, swollen ankles and feet, and the need to urinate more often, especially at night.

Understanding the Symptoms

The good thing is that we can prevent the chronic stage of renal disease by identifying the early signs of any form of kidney damage. Even when a person feels minor changes in his body, he should consult an expert to confirm if it might lead to something serious. The following are a few of the early symptoms of renal damage:

- Tiredness or drowsiness

- Muscle cramps

- Loss of appetite

- Changes in the frequency of urination

- Swelling of hands and feet

- **A feeling of itchiness**
- **Numbness**
- **The darkness of skin**
- **Trouble in sleeping**
- **Shortness of breath**
- **The feeling of nausea or vomiting**

These symptoms can appear in combination with one another. These are general signs of body malfunction, and they should never be ignored. And if they are left unnoticed, they can lead to worsening of the condition and may appear as:

- **Back pain**
- **Abdominal pain**
- **Fever**
- **Rash**
- **Diarrhea**
- **Nosebleeds**
- **Vomiting**

After witnessing any of these symptoms, a person should immediately consult a health expert and prepare himself or herself for the required lifestyle changes.

The Five Stages of Kidney Disease

Chronic kidney disease is categorized into five stages, each one characterized by a certain degree of damage done to the kidneys and rate of glomerular filtration, which is the rate at which filtration takes place in the kidneys. These help us understand just how well the kidneys are functioning.

Stage 1

The first stage is the least severe and actually comes close to a healthy state of your kidneys. Most people will never be aware if they have entered stage 1 of chronic kidney disease, or CKD. In many cases, if people discover stage 1 CKD, then it is because they were being tested for diabetes or high blood pressure. Otherwise, people can find out about stage 1 CKD if they discover protein or blood in the urine, signs of kidney damage in an ultrasound, a computerized tomography (CT) scan or through magnetic resonance imaging (MRI). If people have a family history of polycystic kidney disease (PKD), then there are chances that they might have CKD as well.

Stage 2

In this stage, there is a mild decrease in the glomerular filtration rate. People don't usually notice any symptoms at this stage as well. The reasons for discovering any signs of CKD is the same as the reasons provided in stage 1.

So, what's the difference between stage 1 and stage 2? It all lies in the glomerular filtration rate, or GFR for short. The GFR is measured in milliliters/minute.

In stage 1, the glomerular filtration rate (GFR) is around 90 ml/min. The normal range of the GFR is from 90 ml/min to 120 ml/min. So, as you can see, stage 1 CKD shows a GFR at the lower end of the range. Because it falls so close to a normal rate, it easily goes unnoticed. At stage 2, the GFR falls to between 60-89 ml/min. You might become concerned with the range stage 2 falls in, but your kidneys are actually resilient. Even if they are not functioning at 100 percent, your kidneys are capable of doing a good job. So good that you might not notice anything was out of the ordinary.

Even though the differences between stage 1 and 2 are minuscule, they cannot be combined because the chances of someone showing certain symptoms of CKD when in stage 2 are greater.

Stage 3

At this stage, the kidneys suffer moderate damage. To properly gauge the level of damage, this stage is further divided into two: stage 3A and stage 3B. The reason for the division is because even though the severity of the disease worsens from 3A to 3B, the damage to the kidneys are still within moderate levels.

Each of the divisions is characterized by their GFR.

- 3A has a GFR between 45-59 ml/min

- 3B has a GFR between 30-44 ml/min

When patients reach stage 3, they begin to experience other symptoms of CKD, which include the below:

- Increase in fatigue

- Shortness of breath and swelling of extremities, also called edema

- Slight kidney pain, where the pain is felt in the lower back area

- Change in the color of urine

Stage 4

At stage 4, the kidney disease becomes severe. The GFR falls down to 15-30 ml/min. As the waste buildup increases the patient might experience nausea and vomiting, a buildup of urea in the blood that could cause bad breath, and find themselves having trouble doing everyday tasks such as reading a newspaper or trying to write up an email.

It is important to see a nephrologist (a doctor who specializes in kidney problems) when the patient reaches stage 4.

Stage 5

At stage 5, the kidneys have a GFR of less than 15 ml/min. This is a truly low rate that causes the waste buildup to reach a critical point. The organs have reached an advanced stage of CKD, causing them to lose almost all their abilities in order to function normally.

CHAPTER 2.
RENAL DIET GUIDELINES

If you have been diagnosed with kidney dysfunction, a proper diet is necessary for controlling the amount of toxic waste in the bloodstream. When toxic waste piles up in the system along with increased fluid, chronic inflammation occurs and we have a much higher chance of developing cardiovascular, bone, metabolic or other health issues.

A renal diet is an eating plan exercised to help minimize waste products' levels in the blood. The renal diet is designed to cause as little work or stress on the kidneys as possible, while still providing energy and the high nutrients the body needs.

A renal diet follows several fundamental guidelines. The first is that it must be a balanced, healthy, and sustainable diet, rich in natural grains, vitamins, fibers, carbohydrates, omega 3 fats, and fluids. Proteins should be adequate, but not excessive.

Accumulates in the blood are kept to a minimum. Blood electrolyte levels are monitored regularly, and the diet is corrected. It is essential to follow specific advice from your doctor and dietitian.

Daily protein intake is essential to rebuild tissues but needs to be kept to a minimum. Superfluous proteins need to be broken down by the body into nitrates and carbs. Nitrates are not employed by the body and have to be excreted via the kidneys.

Carbohydrates are a very important source of energy and should be taken in adequate amounts. Whole grains are the best. Avoid highly refined carbohydrates.

Table salt ought to be limited to cooking only. Excess salt overworks the kidneys and causes fluid retention. Salty foods like processed meats, lots of foods, sausages, and snacks should be avoided.

Phosphorus is essential for the body to function, but dialysis can't remove it, so amounts need to be monitored, and intake should be restricted though not eliminated completely.

Foods, like dairy products, darker drinks such as colas and legumes, have high phosphorus content. If levels of this increase in the blood, foods high in potassium such as citrus fruits and dark, leafy green lettuce, carrots or apricots might have to be restricted.

Omega 3 fats are a significant part of any healthy diet. Fish is an excellent source. Omega fats are important for the body. Avoid trans-fats or hydrolyzed fats.

Fluids should be enough but might need to be limited in cases of fluid retention.

A healthy renal diet can help keep kidney function for longer. The main differences between a renal diet and any nutritious diet plan are the limitations placed on protein and table salt ingestion. Restrictions on fluids and potassium might become necessary as signs and symptoms of accumulation become evident.

For people with diabetes who also suffer from kidney disease, there is a food strategy or diet. Over fifty percent of chronic kidney disease sufferers are people that have diabetes, indicating the necessity for them to stick to the diabetic diet.

In several cases, this diet is prepared and is effective in different phases of this disease. There are also instances where the diet is created for diabetics hoping to avoid renal disorder. Sufferers of diabetes and kidney problems have trouble eating the proper food.

The aim of a diabetic's meal plan would be to get the blood within the safe selection. This may be carried out just by having meals frequently on a daily basis, not missing any, and eating carbohydrate foods that are low glycemic.

Consuming a number of such carbohydrates at every meal can assist the body in maintaining a moderate blood sugar level, becoming neither too high nor too low.

Low glycemic foods include brown rice, sweet potatoes, and whole-grain bread. But if it is a renal diet for diabetics, whole-grain bread and sweet potatoes ought not to be used since they're rich in potassium.

For people with kidney issues, they should eat less of these foods full of potassium, phosphorus and sodium. A blood sugar-lowering diet for people with diabetes can be a diet suitable for renal issues. Patients need to check labels since sodium is common in several foods.

For clients with kidney problems, dietitians advise against the consumption of diet pops of java because such drinks contain sodium.

On a diabetic-renal meal plan, unsweetened teas, water and diet sodas are allowed. When it comes to vegetables, broccoli, cauliflower, beets, eggplant, and cabbage are usually recommended because of their abundant vitamin content and very low carbohydrate and potassium content. Meats that are rich in sodium, such as organ meats, sausage, and bacon, ought not to be taken.

Since canned vegetables contain lots of sodium, it is necessary to choose raw vegetables and steer clear of the canned variety. Furthermore, raw vegetables are more nutritious, considering their vitamins.

It is recommended that diabetics learn from certified nutritionists the foods that they need to eat or avoid.

However, all forms of renal diet have one thing in common, which is to improve your renal functions, bring some relief to your kidneys, as well as prevent kidneys disease in patients with numerous risk factors, altogether improving your overall health and wellbeing. The grocery list we have provided should help you get ahold of which groceries you should introduce to your diet and which groups of food should be avoided in order to improve your kidneys' performance, so you can start from shopping for your new lifestyle.

You don't need to shop for many different types of groceries all at once as it is always better to use fresh produce, although frozen food also makes a good alternative when fresh fruit and vegetables are not available.

As far as the renal diet we are recommending in our guide, this form of kidney-friendly dietary regimen offers a solution in form of low-sodium and low-potassium meals and groceries, which is why we are also offering simple and easy renal diet recipes in our guide. By following a dietary plan compiled for all stages of renal system failure unless the doctor recommends a different treatment by allowing or expelling some of the groceries, we have listed in our ultimate grocery list for renal patients.

Before we get to cooking and changing your lifestyle from the very core with the idea of improving your health, we want you to get familiar with renal diet basics and find out exactly what his diet is based on while you already know what is the very core solution found in renal diet – helping you improve your kidney's health by lowering sodium and potassium intake.

The best way of getting familiar with the renal diet and basics of this dietary regimen is to take a look at the most commonly asked questions that extend the answer to the question What is the renal diet?

The Benefits of Renal Diet

Renal diets help people with kidney disease increase their quality of life.

Other types of food may be harmful to kidneys infected with a disease, so you need to make sure you have a sound knowledge of the infection and how it affects the body.

You don't want kidney disease, but there are ways to boost your well-being by changing your diet. In reality, renal diets help you manage your health and reduce kidney disease.

You need to remember—changing your diet won't heal everybody, but it can help everyone. This doesn't mean a diet is a cure-all, so don't think of this article as medical advice; it's more of a guide.

Your doctor can provide more guidance than this does and should always be informed or notified of any improvement in your condition.

If you have kidney problems, it's essential to regulate your health to help you feel better. There are entire books devoted to renal diets, or you can check with a registered dietitian for recommendations. Using a Kindle or iPad, you can even download and access these books instantly.

Dietitians have experience working with those with kidney problems and can give some general do's and don'ts to follow, such as: control potassium intake—fruits like strawberries and apples are low in potassium, along with vegetables like cauliflower, cabbage and broccoli.

Track your phosphorous consumption—-creamers, pasta, cereals and rice are on the OK list.

Restrict liquid intake to 48 oz. This is the recommended level of liquid per day for renal diets. be sure to count fluid in items like oranges, ice cream etc.

Track your salt intake—you'll need to be a tag reader to make sure you keep your salt intake low—-know what you're putting in your body and what it might contain.

Regulate your protein intake—maintain 5-7 ounces. Use egg replacements instead of normal eggs as a good technique for low protein consumption.

If you choose to use a dietitian, they can point you precisely to what you should and shouldn't consume, and why. Being aware of the effect food has on your body is important and can help you feel good every day. Also, this design is not an alternative to clinical guidelines. Yet renal diets help most kidney disease sufferers to become and stay healthier.

CHAPTER 3.
31-DAYS PLAN

Day	Breakfast	Lunch	Dinner	Snacks
1	Chessy Scrambled Egg with Fries Herbs	Dolmas Wrap	Eggplant and Red Pepper Soup	Moo-Less Chocolate Mousse
2	Turkey and Spinach Scramble on Melba Toast	Salad al Tonno	Seafood Casserole	Baked Carrots
3	Vegetable Omelet	Arlecchino Rice Salad	Ground Beef and Rice Soup	Cranberry & Apple Coleslaw
4	Mexican Style Burritos	Greek Salad	Couscous Burgers	Roasted Beet & Canned Sardine Salad
5	Blueberry Muffins	Sauteed Chickpea and Lentil Mix	Baked Flounder	Chicken & Zucchini Hot Salad
6	Bulgur, Couscous and Buckwheat Cereal	Buffalo Chicken Lettuce Wraps	Persian Chicken	Tuna Salad
7	Sweet Pancakes	Crazy Japanese Potato and Beef Croquettes	Pork Souvlaki	Ginger-Lime Grilled Shrimp
8	Breakfast Smoothie	Spicy Chili Crackers	Pork Meatloaf	Seafood Jambalaya
9	Buckwheat and Grapefruit Porridge	Golden Eggplant Fries	Chicken Stew	Kale Chips
10	Egg and Veggie Muffins	Traditional Black Bean Chili	Beef Chili	Tortilla Chips
11	Berry Chia with Yogurt	Very Wild Mushroom Pilaf	Shrimp Paella	Corn Bread
12	Arugula Eggs with Chili Peppers	Green Palak Paneer	Salmon & Pesto Salad	Vegetable Rolls
13	Breakfast Skillet	Sporty Baby Carrots	Baked Fennel & Garlic Sea Bass	Frittata with Penne

14	Eggs in Tomato Rings	Saucy Garlic Greens	Lemon, Garlic & Cilantro Tuna and Rice	Buffalo Cauliflower Bites with Dairy Free Ranch Dressing
15	Eggplant Chicken Sandwich	Garden Salad	Cod & Green Bean Risotto	Baked Cream Cheese Crab Dip
16	Eggplant Caprese	Spicy Cabbage Dish	Sardine Fish Cakes	Philly Cheesesteak Stuffed Mushrooms
17	Chorizo Bowl with Corn	Extreme Balsamic Chicken	Cajun Catfish	Greek Cookies
18	Panzanella Salad	Enjoyable Spinach and Bean Medley	4-Ingredients Salmon Fillet	Ham and Dill Pickle Bites
19	Panzanella Salad	Tantalizing Cauliflower and Dill Mash	Spanish Cod in Sauce	Easy Flavored Potatoes Mix
20	Strawberry Muesli	Secret Asian Green Beans	Fish Shakshuka	Moo-Less Chocolate Mousse
21	Poached Asparagus and Egg	Dolmas Wrap	Eggplant and Red Pepper Soup	Baked Carrots
22	Apple Turnover	Salad al Tonno	Seafood Casserole	Cranberry & Apple Coleslaw
23	Egg Drop Soup	Arlecchino Rice Salad	Ground Beef and Rice Soup	Roasted Beet & Canned Sardine Salad
24	Chessy Scrambled Egg with Fries Herbs	Greek Salad	Couscous Burgers	Chicken & Zucchini Hot Salad
25	Turkey and Spinach Scramble on Melba Toast	Sauteed Chickpea and Lentil Mix	Baked Flounder	Tuna Salad
26	Vegetable Omelet	Buffalo Chicken Lettuce Wraps	Persian Chicken	Ginger-Lime Grilled Shrimp

27	Mexican Style Burritos	Crazy Japanese Potato and Beef Croquettes	Pork Souvlaki	Seafood Jambalaya
28	Blueberry Muffins	Spicy Chili Crackers	Pork Meatloaf	Kale Chips
29	Bulgur, Couscous and Buckwheat Cereal	Golden Eggplant Fries	Chicken Stew	Tortilla Chips
30	Sweet Pancakes	Traditional Black Bean Chili	Beef Chili	Corn Bread
31	Apple Onion Omelet	Chicken Wild Rice	Pepper Bacon	Beef Brisket

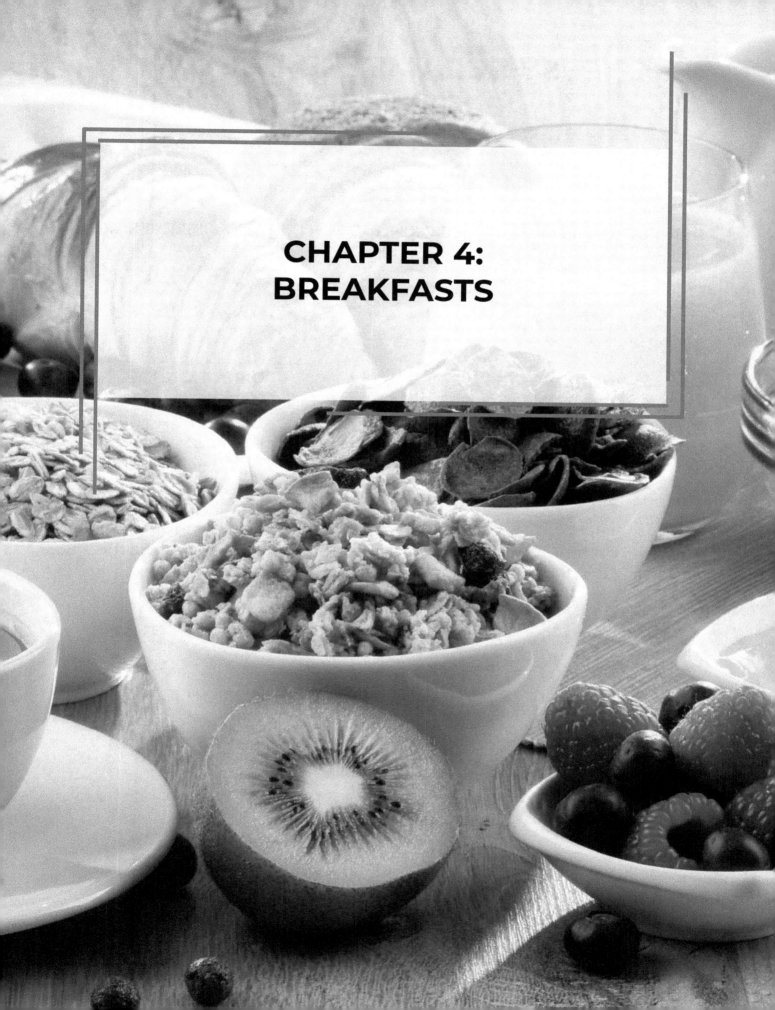

CHAPTER 4:
BREAKFASTS

1. CHEESY SCRAMBLED EGGS WITH FRESH HERBS

PREPARATION: 15 MIN   **COOKING: 10 MIN**   **SERVES: 4**

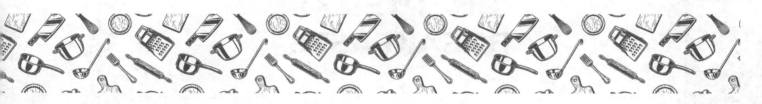

INGREDIENTS

- Eggs – 3
- Egg whites – 2
- Cream cheese – ½ cup
- Unsweetened rice milk – ¼ cup
- Chopped scallion – 1 Tbsp. green part only
- Chopped fresh tarragon – 1 Tbsp.
- Unsalted butter – 2 Tbsps.
- Ground black pepper to taste

DIRECTIONS

1. In a bowl, whisk the eggs, cream cheese, rice milk, scallions, and tarragon until mixed and smooth.
2. Melt the butter in a skillet.
3. Pour in the egg mixture and cook, stirring, for 5 minutes or until the eggs are thick and curds creamy.
4. Season with pepper and serve.

Nutritions: *Calories: 221, Fat: 19g, Carb: 3g, Phosphorus: 119mg, Potassium: 140mg, Sodium: 193mg, Protein: 8g*

2. TURKEY AND SPINACH SCRAMBLE ON MELBA TOAST

PREPARATION: 2 MIN

COOKING: 15 MIN

SERVES: 2

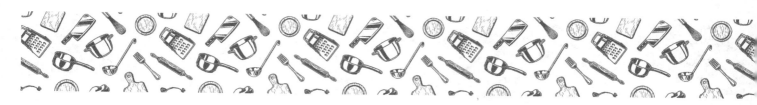

INGREDIENTS

- Extra virgin olive oil – 1 tsp
- Raw spinach – 1 cup
- Garlic – ½ clove, minced
- Nutmeg – 1 tsp. grated
- Cooked and diced turkey breast – 1 cup
- Melba toast – 4 slices
- Balsamic vinegar – 1 tsp.

DIRECTIONS

1. Heat a skillet over a medium temperature and add oil.
2. Add turkey and heat through for 6 to 8 minutes.
3. Add spinach, garlic, and nutmeg and stir-fry for 6 minutes more.
4. Plate up the Melba toast and top with spinach and turkey scramble.
5. Drizzle with balsamic vinegar and serve.

Nutritions: *Calories: 301, Fat: 19g, Carb: 12g, Phosphorus: 215mg, Potassium: 269mg, Sodium: 360mg, Protein: 19g*

3. VEGETABLE OMELET

PREPARATION: 15 MIN

COOKING: 10 MIN

SERVES: 3

INGREDIENTS

- Egg whites – 4
- Egg – 1
- Chopped fresh parsley – 2 Tbsps.
- Water – 2 Tbsps.
- Olive oil spray
- Chopped and boiled red bell pepper – ½ cup
- Chopped scallion – ¼ cup, both green and white parts
- Ground black pepper

DIRECTIONS

1. Whisk together the egg, egg whites, parsley, and water until well blended. Set aside.
2. Spray the skillet with oil and place over medium heat.
3. Sauté the peppers and scallion for 3 minutes or until softened.
4. Pour the egg mixture into the skillet over vegetables and cook, swirling the skillet, for 2 minutes or until the edges start to set. Cook until set.
5. Season with black pepper and serve.

Nutritions: *Calories: 77, Fat: 3g, Carb: 2g, Phosphorus: 67mg, Potassium: 194mg, Sodium: 229mg, Protein: 12g*

4. MEXICAN STYLE BURRITOS

PREPARATION: 5 MIN

COOKING: 15 MIN

SERVES: 2

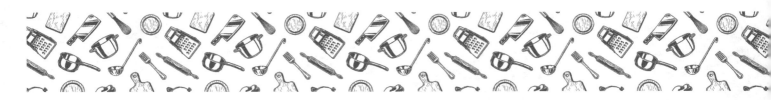

INGREDIENTS

- Olive oil – 1 Tbsp.
- Corn tortillas – 2
- Red onion – ¼ cup, chopped
- Red bell peppers – ¼ cup, chopped
- Red chili – ½, deseeded and chopped
- Eggs – 2
- Juice of 1 lime
- Cilantro – 1 Tbsp. chopped

DIRECTIONS

1. Turn the broiler to medium heat and place the tortillas underneath for 1 to 2 minutes on each side or until lightly toasted.
2. Remove and keep the broiler on.
3. Heat oil in a skillet and sauté onion, chili and bell peppers for 5 to 6 minutes or until soft.
4. Crack eggs over the top of the onions and peppers and place skillet under the broiler for 5 to 6 minutes or until the eggs are cooked.
5. Serve half the eggs and vegetables on top of each tortilla and sprinkle with cilantro and lime juice to serve.

Nutritions: *Calories: 202, Fat: 13g, Carb: 19g, Phosphorus: 184mg, Potassium: 233mg, Sodium: 77mg, Protein: 9g*

5. BLUEBERRY MUFFINS

PREPARATION: 15 MIN

COOKING: 30 MIN

SERVES: 12

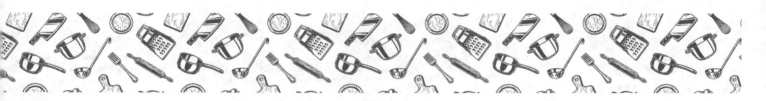

INGREDIENTS

- Unsweetened rice milk – 2 cups
- Apple cider vinegar – 1 Tbsp.
- All-purpose flour – 3 ½ cups
- Granulated sugar – 1 cup
- Baking soda substitute – 1 Tbsp.
- Ground cinnamon – 1 tsp.
- Ground nutmeg – ½ tsp.
- Pinch ground ginger
- Canola oil – ½ cup
- Pure vanilla extract – 2 Tbsps.
- Fresh blueberries – 2 ½ cups

DIRECTIONS

1. Preheat the oven to 375F.
2. Line the muffin cups with paper liners. Put aside.
3. In a small bowl, blend rice milk and vinegar. Book for 10 minutes.
4. In a large bowl, mix the sugar, flour, baking soda, cinnamon, nutmeg and ginger until well blended.
5. Add the oil and vanilla to the milk mixture and mix well.
6. Add the milk mixture to the dry ingredients and mix until well blended.
7. Incorporate the blueberries. Evenly pour the muffin dough into the cups.
8. Bake the muffins for 25-30 minutes or until they are golden brown and an inserted toothpick is clean
9. Cool for 15 minutes and serve.

Nutritions: *Calories: 331, Fat: 11g, Carb: 52g, Phosphorus: 90mg, Potassium: 89mg, Sodium: 35mg, Protein: 6g*

6. BULGUR, COUSCOUS AND BUCKWHEAT CEREAL

PREPARATION: 10 MIN   **COOKING: 25 MIN**   **SERVES: 4**

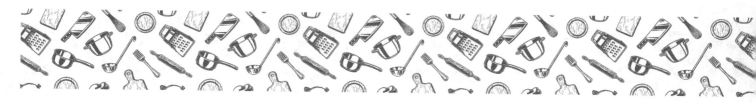

INGREDIENTS

- Water – 2 ¼ cups
- Vanilla rice milk – 1 ¼ cups
- Uncooked bulgur – 6 Tbsps.
- Uncooked whole buckwheat – 2 Tbsps.
- Sliced apple – 1 cup
- Plain uncooked couscous – 6 Tbsps.
- Ground cinnamon – ½ tsp.

DIRECTIONS

1. In the saucepan, heat the water and milk over medium heat.
2. Boil, and add the bulgur, buckwheat, and apple.
3. Reduce the heat to low and simmer, occasionally stirring until the bulgur is tender, about 20 to 25 minutes.
4. Remove saucepan from the heat and stir in the couscous and cinnamon.
5. Let saucepan stand, covered, for 10 minutes.
6. Fluff cereal with a fork before serving.

Nutritions: *Calories: 159, Fat: 1g, Carb: 34g, Phosphorus: 130mg, Potassium: 116mg, Sodium: 33mg, Protein: 4g*

7. SWEET PANCAKES

PREPARATION: 10 MIN

COOKING: 5 MIN

SERVES: 5

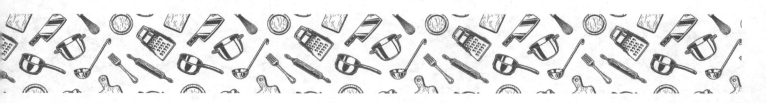

INGREDIENTS

- All-purpose flour – 1 cup
- Granulated sugar – 1 Tbsp.
- Baking powder – 2 tsps.
- Egg whites – 2
- Almond milk - 1 cup
- Olive oil - 2 Tbsps.
- Maple extract – 1 Tbsp.

DIRECTIONS

1. Blend the flour and baking powder in a bowl.
2. Make a well in the center and place on one side.
3. In another bowl, mix the egg whites, milk, oil, and maple extract.
4. Add the egg mixture to the well and gently mix until a batter is formed.
5. Heat skillet over medium heat.
6. Add 1/5 of the batter to the pan and cook 2 minutes on each side or until the pancake is golden.
7. Repeat with the remaining batter and serve.

Nutritions: *Calories: 178, Fat: 6g, Carb: 25g, Phosphorus: 116mg, Potassium: 126mg, Sodium: 297mg, Protein: 6g*

8. BREAKFAST SMOOTHIE

PREPARATION: 15 MIN

COOKING: 0 MIN

SERVES: 2

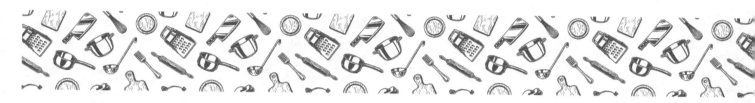

INGREDIENTS

- Frozen blueberries – 1 cup
- Pineapple chunks – ½ cup
- English cucumber – ½ cup
- Apple – ½
- Water – ½ cup

DIRECTIONS

1. Put the pineapple, blueberries, cucumber, apple, and water in a blender and blend until thick and smooth.
2. Pour into 2 glasses and serve.

Nutritions: *Calories: 87, Fat: g, Carb: 22g, Phosphorus: 28mg, Potassium: 192mg, Sodium: 3mg, Protein: 0.7g*

9. BUCKWHEAT AND GRAPEFRUIT PORRIDGE

PREPARATION: 5 MIN

COOKING: 20 MIN

SERVES: 2

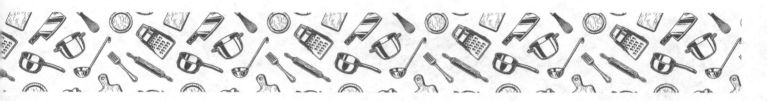

INGREDIENTS

- Buckwheat – ½ cup
- Grapefruit – ¼, chopped
- Honey – 1 Tbsp.
- Almond milk – 1 ½ cups
- Water – 2 cups

DIRECTIONS

1. Boil water on the stove. Add the buckwheat and place the lid on the pan.
2. Lower heat slightly and simmer for 7 to 10 minutes, checking to ensure water does not dry out.
3. When most of the water is absorbed, remove and set aside for 5 minutes.
4. Drain any excess water from the pan and stir in almond milk, heating through for 5 minutes.
5. Add the honey and grapefruit.
6. Serve.

Nutritions: *Calories: 231, Fat: 4g, Carb: 43g, Phosphorus: 165mg, Potassium: 370mg, Sodium: 135mg*

10. EGG AND VEGGIE MUFFINS

PREPARATION: 15 MIN

COOKING: 20 MIN

SERVES: 4

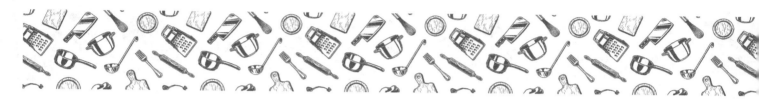

INGREDIENTS

- Cooking spray
- Eggs – 4
- Unsweetened rice milk – 2 Tbsp.
- Sweet onion – ½, chopped
- Red bell pepper – ½, chopped
- Pinch red pepper flakes
- Pinch ground black pepper

DIRECTIONS

1. Preheat the oven to 350F.
2. Spray 4 muffin pans with cooking spray. Set aside.
3. In a medium bowl, whisk together the milk, eggs, onion, red pepper, parsley, red pepper flakes, and black pepper until mixed.
4. Pour the egg mixture into prepared muffin pans.
5. Bake until the muffins are puffed and golden, about 18 to 20 minutes.
6. serve

Nutritions: *Calories: 84, Fat: 5g, Carb: 3g, Phosphorus: 110mg, Potassium: 117mg, Sodium: 75mg, Protein: 7g*

11. BERRY CHIA WITH YOGURT

PREPARATION: 35 MIN

COOKING: 5 MIN

SERVES: 4

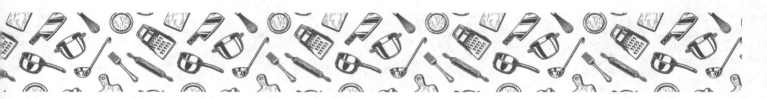

INGREDIENTS

- ½ cup chia seeds, dried
- 2 cup Plain yogurt
- 1/3 cup strawberries, chopped
- ¼ cup blackberries
- ¼ cup raspberries
- 4 teaspoons Splenda

DIRECTIONS

1. Mix up together Plain yogurt with Splenda, and chia seeds.
2. Transfer the mixture into the serving ramekins (jars) and leave for 35 minutes.
3. After this, add blackberries, raspberries, and strawberries. Mix up the meal well.
4. Serve it immediately or store in the fridge up to 2 days.

Nutritions: *Calories 257, Fat 10.3, Fiber 11, Carbs 27.2, Protein 12*

12. ARUGULA EGGS WITH CHILI PEPPERS

PREPARATION: 7 MIN

COOKING: 10 MIN

SERVES: 4

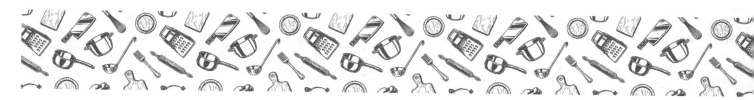

INGREDIENTS

- 2 cups arugula, chopped
- 3 eggs, beaten
- ½ chili pepper, chopped
- 1 tablespoon butter
- 1 oz Parmesan, grated

DIRECTIONS

1. Toss butter in the skillet and melt it.
2. Add arugula and saute it over the medium heat for 5 minutes. Stir it from time to time.
3. Meanwhile, mix up together Parmesan, chili pepper, and eggs.
4. Pour the egg mixture over the arugula and scramble well.
5. Cook the breakfast for 5 minutes more over the medium heat.

Nutritions: *Calories 98, Fat 7.8, Fiber 0.2, Carbs 0.9, Protein 6.7*

13. BREAKFAST SKILLET

PREPARATION: 7 MIN

COOKING: 25 MIN

SERVES: 5

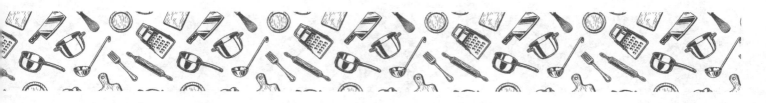

INGREDIENTS

- 1 cup cauliflower, chopped
- 1 tablespoon olive oil
- ½ red onion, diced
- 1 tablespoon Plain yogurt
- ½ teaspoon ground black pepper
- 1 teaspoon dried cilantro
- 1 teaspoon dried oregano
- 1 bell pepper, chopped
- 1/3 cup milk
- ½ teaspoon Za'atar
- 1 tablespoon lemon juice
- 1 russet potato, chopped

DIRECTIONS

1. Pour olive oil in the skillet and preheat it.
2. Add chopped russet potato and roast it for 5 minutes.
3. After this, add cauliflower, ground black pepper, cilantro, oregano, and bell pepper.
4. Roast the mixture for 10 minutes over the medium heat.
5. Then add milk, Za'atar, and Plain Yogurt. Stir it well.
6. Saute the mixture 10 minutes.
7. Top the cooked meal with diced red onion and sprinkle with lemon juice.
8. It is recommended to serve the breakfast hot.

Nutritions: *Calories 112, Fat 3.4, Fiber 2.6, Carbs 18.1, Protein 3.1*

14. EGGS IN TOMATO RINGS

PREPARATION: 8 MIN

COOKING: 5 MIN

SERVES: 2

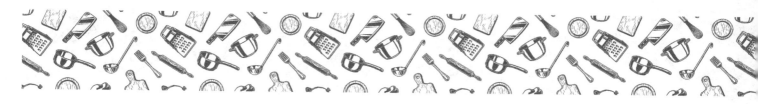

INGREDIENTS

- 1 tomato
- 2 eggs
- ¼ teaspoon chili flakes
- ¾ teaspoon salt
- ½ teaspoon butter

DIRECTIONS

1. Trim the tomato and slice it into 2 rings.
2. Remove the tomato flesh.
3. Toss butter in the skillet and melt it.
4. Then arrange the tomato rings.
5. Crack the eggs in the tomato rings. Sprinkle them with salt and chili flakes.
6. Cook the eggs for 4 minutes over the medium heat with the closed lid.
7. Transfer the cooked eggs into the serving plates with the help of the spatula.

Nutritions: *Calories 77, Fat 5.4, Fiber 0.4, Carbs 1.6, Protein 5.8*

15. SAUSAGE CASSEROLE

PREPARATION: 10 MIN

COOKING: 50 MIN

SERVES: 8

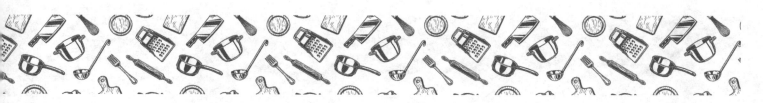

INGREDIENTS

- 12 eggs
- 1 lb. ground Italian sausage
- 2 1/2 tomatoes, sliced
- 3 tbsp coconut flour
- 1/4 cup coconut milk
- 2 small zucchinis, shredded
- Pepper
- Salt

DIRECTIONS

1. Preheat the oven to 350 F.
2. Cook sausage in a pan until brown.
3. Transfer sausage to a mixing bowl.
4. Add coconut flour, milk, eggs, zucchini, pepper, and salt. Stir well.
5. Add eggs and whisk to combine.
6. Transfer bowl mixture into the casserole dish and top with tomato slices.
7. Bake for 50 minutes.
8. Serve and enjoy.

Nutritions: *Calories 305, Fat 21.8 g, Carbohydrates 6.3 g, Sugar 3.3 g, Protein 19.6 g, Cholesterol 286 mg*

16. BAKED CURRIED APPLE OATMEAL CUPS

PREPARATION: 10 MIN

COOKING: 20 MIN

SERVES: 6

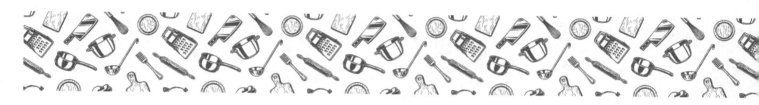

INGREDIENTS

- 3½ cups old-fashioned oats
- 3 tablespoons brown sugar
- 2 teaspoons of your preferred curry powder
- 1/8 teaspoon salt
- 1 cup unsweetened almond milk
- 1 cup unsweetened applesauce
- 1 teaspoon vanilla
- ½ cup chopped walnuts

DIRECTIONS

1. Preheat the oven to 375°.Spray a cup muffin tin with baking spray then set aside.
2. Combine the oats, brown sugar, curry powder, and salt, and mix in a medium bowl.
3. Mix together the milk, applesauce, and vanilla in a small bowl,
4. Stir the liquid ingredients into the dry ingredients and mix until just combined. Stir in the walnuts.
5. Using a scant 1/3 cup for each divide the mixture among the muffin cups.
6. Bake this for 18 to 20 minutes until the oatmeal is firm. Serve.

Nutritions: *Calories: 296; Total fat: 10g; Saturated fat: 1g; Sodium: 84mg; Phosphorus: 236mg; Potassium: 289mg; Carbohydrates: 45g; Fiber: 6g; Protein: 8g; Sugar: 11g*

17. PANZANELLA SALAD

PREPARATION: 10 MIN

COOKING: 5 MIN

SERVES: 4

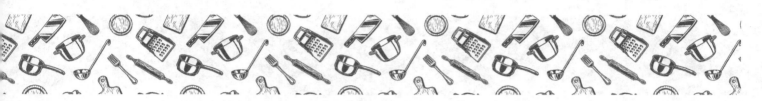

INGREDIENTS

- 3 tomatoes, chopped
- 2 cucumbers, chopped
- 1 red onion, sliced
- 2 red bell peppers, chopped
- ¼ cup fresh cilantro, chopped
- 1 tablespoon capers
- 1 oz whole-grain bread, chopped
- 1 tablespoon canola oil
- ½ teaspoon minced garlic
- 1 tablespoon Dijon mustard
- 1 teaspoon olive oil
- 1 teaspoon lime juice

DIRECTIONS

1. Pour canola oil in the skillet and bring it to boil.
2. Add chopped bread and roast it until crunchy (3-5 minutes).
3. Meanwhile, in the salad bowl combine together sliced red onion, cucumbers, tomatoes, bell peppers, cilantro, capers, and mix up gently.
4. Make the dressing: mix up together lime juice, olive oil, Dijon mustard, and minced garlic.
5. Transfer the dressing over the salad and stir it directly before serving.

Nutritions: *Calories 136, Fat 5.7, Fiber 4.1, Carbs 20.2, Protein 4.1*

18. SHRIMP BRUSCHETTA

PREPARATION: 15 MIN

COOKING: 10 MIN

SERVES: 4

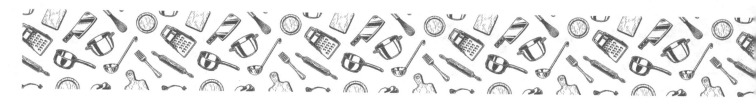

INGREDIENTS

- 13 oz shrimps, peeled
- 1 tablespoon tomato sauce
- ½ teaspoon Splenda
- ¼ teaspoon garlic powder
- 1 teaspoon fresh parsley, chopped
- ½ teaspoon olive oil
- 1 teaspoon lemon juice
- 4 whole-grain bread slices
- 1 cup water, for cooking

DIRECTIONS

1. Pour the water in a pot and bring it to boil.
2. Add shrimps and boil them over the high heat for 5 minutes.
3. After this, drain shrimps and chill them to the room temperature.
4. Mix up together shrimps with Splenda, garlic powder, tomato sauce, and fresh parsley.
5. Add lemon juice and stir gently.
6. Preheat the oven to 360F.
7. Brush bread with olive oil and bake for 3 minutes.
8. Then place the shrimp mixture on the bread. Bruschetta is cooked.

Nutritions: *Calories 199, Fat 3.7, Fiber 2.1, Carbs 15.3, Protein 24.1*

19. STRAWBERRY MUESLI

PREPARATION: 10 MIN

COOKING: 30 MIN

SERVES: 4

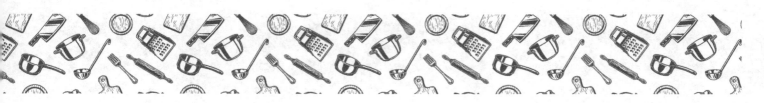

INGREDIENTS

- 2 cups Greek yogurt
- 1 ½ cup strawberries, sliced
- 1 ½ cup Muesli
- 4 teaspoon maple syrup
- ¾ teaspoon ground cinnamon

DIRECTIONS

1. Put Greek yogurt in the food processor.
2. Add 1 cup of strawberries, maple syrup, and ground cinnamon.
3. Blend the ingredients until you get smooth mass.
4. Transfer the yogurt mass in the serving bowls.
5. Add Muesli and stir well.
6. Leave the meal for 30 minutes in the fridge.
7. After this, decorate it with remaining sliced strawberries.

Nutritions: *Calories 149, Fat 2.6, Fiber 3.6, Carbs 21.6, Protein 12*

20. POACHED ASPARAGUS AND EGG

PREPARATION: 3 MIN

COOKING: 15 MIN

SERVES: 1

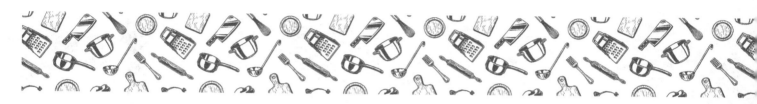

INGREDIENTS

- 1 egg
- 4 spears asparagus
- Water

DIRECTIONS

1. Half-fill a deep saucepan with water set over high heat. Let the water come to a boil.
2. Dip asparagus spears in water. Cook until they turn a shade brighter, about 3 minutes. Remove from saucepan and drain on paper towels. Keep warm. Lightly season prior to serving.
3. Using a slotted spoon, gently lower egg into boiling water. Cook for only 4 minutes. Remove from pan immediately. Place on egg holder.
4. Slice off the top. The egg should still be fluid inside.
5. Place asparagus spears on a small plate and serve egg on the side. Dip asparagus into the egg and eat while warm.

Nutritions: *Calories 178, Carbs 1g, Fat 13g, Protein 7.72g, Potassium (K) 203 mg, Sodium (Na) 71 mg, Phosphorus 124 mg*

21. APPLE TURNOVER

PREPARATION: 10 MIN

COOKING: 15 MIN

SERVES: 8

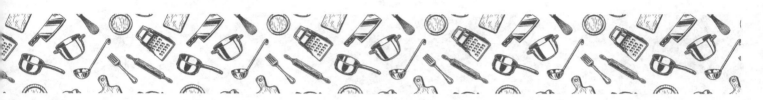

INGREDIENTS

For the turnovers:
- ½ tsp. cinnamon powder
- All-purpose flour
- ½ cup unwashed palm sugar
- 1 tbsp. almond flour
- 1 frozen puff pastry
- 4 peeled, cored and diced baking apples.

For the egg wash:
- 2 tbsps. Water
- 1 whisked egg white

DIRECTIONS

1. To make the filling: combine almond flour, cinnamon powder and palm sugar until these resemble coarse meal. Toss in diced apples until well coated. Set aside.
2. On a coated surface, roll out the puff pastry until ¼ inch thin. Slice into 8 pieces of 4" x 4" squares.
3. Divide the prepared apples into 8 equal portions. Spoon on individual puff pastry squares. Fold in half diagonally. Press edges to seal.
4. Place each filled pastry on a baking tray lined with parchment paper. Make sure there is ample space between pastries.
5. Freeze for at least 20 minutes, or until ready to bake.
6. Preheat oven to 400°F for 10 minutes.
7. Brush frozen pastries with egg wash. Place in the hot oven, and cook for 12 to 15 minutes, or until they turn golden brown all over.
8. Remove baking tray from oven immediately. Cool slightly for easier handling.
9. Place 1 apple turnover on a plate. Serve warm.

Nutritions: *Protein 3.81g, Potassium (K) 151 mg, Sodium (Na) 86 mg, Carbs 35.75g, Calories 285, Fat 14.78g, Phosphorus 43.4mg*

22. EGG DROP SOUP

PREPARATION: 5 MIN

COOKING: 10 MIN

SERVES: 4

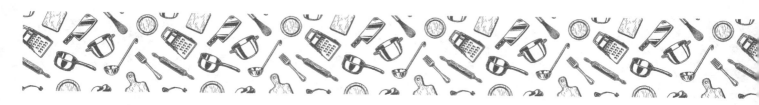

INGREDIENTS

- ¼ cup minced fresh chives
- 4 cups unsalted vegetable stock
- 4 whisked eggs

DIRECTIONS

1. Pour unsalted vegetable stock into the oven set over high heat. Bring to a boil. Turn heat to the lowest heat setting.
2. Pour in the eggs. Stir continuously until ribbons form into the soup.
3. Turn off the heat immediately. The residual heat will cook eggs through.
4. Cool slightly before ladling the desired amount into individual bowls. Garnish with a pinch of parsley, if using. Serve immediately.

Nutritions: *Calories 32, Carbs 0g, Fat 2 g, Protein 5.57g, Potassium (K) 67 mg, Sodium (Na) 63 mg, Phosphorus 36.1mg*

23. EGGS IN TOMATO RINGS

PREPARATION: 8 MIN   COOKING: 5 MIN   SERVES: 2

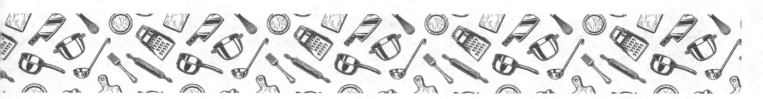

INGREDIENTS

- 1 tomato
- 2 eggs
- ¼ teaspoon chili flakes
- ¾ teaspoon salt
- ½ teaspoon butter

DIRECTIONS

1. Trim the tomato and slice it into 2 rings.
2. Remove the tomato flesh.
3. Toss butter in the skillet and melt it.
4. Then arrange the tomato rings.
5. Crack the eggs in the tomato rings. Sprinkle them with salt and chili flakes.
6. Cook the eggs for 4 minutes over the medium heat with the closed lid.
7. Transfer the cooked eggs into the serving plates with the help of the spatula.

Nutritions: *Calories 77, Fat 5.4g, Fiber 0.4g, Carbs 1.6g, Protein 5.8g*

24. EGGPLANT CHICKEN SANDWICH

PREPARATION: 10 MIN

COOKING: 15 MIN

SERVES: 2

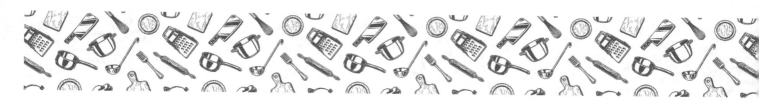

INGREDIENTS

- 1 eggplant, trimmed
- 10 oz chicken fillet
- 1 teaspoon plain yogurt
- ½ teaspoon minced garlic
- 1 tablespoon fresh cilantro, chopped
- 2 lettuce leaves
- 1 teaspoon olive oil
- ½ teaspoon salt
- ½ teaspoon chili pepper
- 1 teaspoon butter

DIRECTIONS

1. Slice the eggplant lengthwise into 4 slices.
2. Rub the eggplant slices with minced garlic and brush with olive oil.
3. Grill the eggplant slices on the preheated to 375F grill for 3 minutes from each side.
4. Meanwhile, rub the chicken fillet with salt and chili pepper.
5. Place it in the skillet and add butter.
6. Roast the chicken for 6 minutes from each side over the medium-high heat.
7. Cool the cooked eggplants gently and spread one side of them with Plain yogurt.
8. Add lettuce leaves and chopped fresh cilantro. After this, slice the cooked chicken fillet and add over the lettuce.
9. Cover it with the remaining sliced eggplant to get the sandwich shape. Pin the sandwich with the toothpick if needed.

Nutritions: *Calories 368, Fat 15.2g, Fiber 8.2g, Carbs 14.2g, Protein 43.5*

25. EGGPLANT CAPRESE

PREPARATION: 15 MIN

COOKING: 13 MIN

SERVES: 3

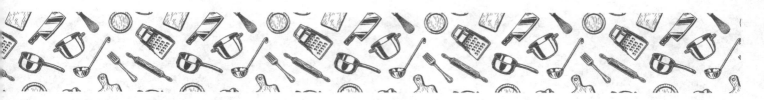

INGREDIENTS

- 1 eggplant, trimmed, sliced
- ½ teaspoon dried basil
- 1 teaspoon salt
- ½ teaspoon ground black pepper
- 2 tomatoes, sliced
- 7 oz Mozzarella, sliced
- 1 teaspoon lemon juice
- 2 tablespoons olive oil

DIRECTIONS

1. Sprinkle the sliced eggplant with salt and leave for 10 minutes or until they give juice.
2. Then sprinkle the sliced eggplants with ground black pepper, lemon juice, and dried basil.
3. Arrange the eggplant, tomato, and sliced Mozzarella one-by-one in the casserole mold.
4. Drizzle it with olive oil and cover with foil.
5. Bake the caprese for 13 minutes.

Nutritions: *Calories 321, Fat 21.5g, Fiber 6.5g, Carbs 14.8, Protein 20.9*

26. CHORIZO BOWL WITH CORN

PREPARATION: 10 MIN

COOKING: 15 MIN

SERVES: 4

INGREDIENTS

- 9 oz chorizo
- 1 tablespoon almond butter
- ½ cup corn kernels
- 1 tomato, chopped
- ¾ cup heavy cream
- 1 teaspoon butter
- ¼ teaspoon chili pepper
- 1 tablespoon dill, chopped

DIRECTIONS

1. Chop the chorizo and place in the skillet.
2. Add almond butter and chili pepper.
3. Roast the chorizo for 3 minutes.
4. After this, add tomato and corn kernels.
5. Add butter and chopped the dill. Mix up the mixture well. Cook for 2 minutes.
6. Close the lid and simmer the meal for 10 minutes over the low heat.
7. Transfer the cooked meal into the serving bowls.

Nutritions: *Calories 422, Fat 36.2g, Fiber 1.2g, Carbs 7.3g, Protein 17.6*

27. ITALIAN BREAKFAST FRITTATA

PREPARATION: 10 MIN

COOKING: 45 MIN

SERVES: 4

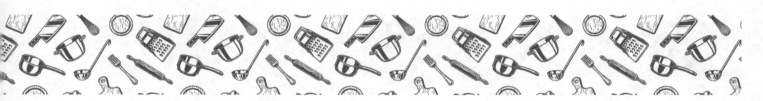

INGREDIENTS

- 2 cups egg whites
- 1/2 cup mozzarella cheese, shredded
- 1 cup cottage cheese, crumbled
- 1/4 cup fresh basil, sliced
- 1/2 cup roasted red peppers, sliced
- Pepper
- Salt

DIRECTIONS

1. Preheat the oven to 375 F.
2. Add ingredients into the bowl and whisk well to combine.
3. Pour frittata mixture into the baking dish and bake for 45 minutes.
4. Slice and serve.

Nutritions: *Calories 131, Fat 2g, Carbohydrates 5g, Sugar 2g, Protein 22g, Cholesterol 6mg*

28. SAUSAGE CHEESE BAKE OMELET

PREPARATION: 10 MIN

COOKING: 45 MIN

SERVES: 8

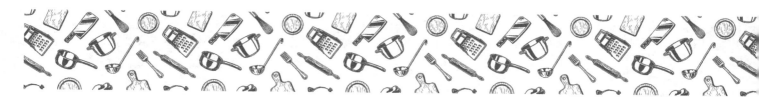

INGREDIENTS

- 16 eggs
- 2 cups cheddar cheese, shredded
- 1/2 cup salsa
- 1 lb ground sausage
- 1 1/2 cups coconut milk
- Pepper
- Salt

DIRECTIONS

1. Preheat the oven to 350 F.
2. Add sausage in a pan and cook until browned. Drain excess fat.
3. In a large bowl, whisk eggs and milk. Stir in cheese, cooked sausage, and salsa.
4. Pour omelet mixture into the baking dish and bake for 45 minutes.
5. Serve and enjoy.

Nutritions: *Calories 360, Fat 24g, Carbohydrates 4g, Sugar 3g, Protein 28g, Cholesterol 400 mg*

29. GREEK EGG SCRAMBLED

PREPARATION: 10 MIN

COOKING: 10 MIN

SERVES: 2

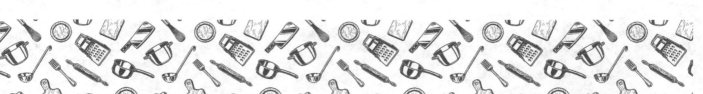

INGREDIENTS

- eggs
- 1/2 cup grape tomatoes, sliced
- 2 tbsp green onions, sliced
- 1 bell pepper, diced
- 1 tbsp olive oil
- 1/4 tsp dried oregano
- 1/2 tbsp capers
- 3 olives, sliced
- Pepper
- Salt

DIRECTIONS

1. Heat the oil in a pan over average heat
2. Add green onions and bell pepper and cook until pepper is softened.
3. Add tomatoes, capers, and olives and cook for 1 minute.
4. Add eggs and stir until eggs are cooked. Season it with oregano, pepper, and salt.
5. Serve and enjoy.

Nutritions: *Calories 230, Fat 17g, Carbohydrates 8g, Sugar 5g, Protein 12g, Cholesterol 325 mg*

30. FETA MINT OMELET

PREPARATION: 10 MIN

COOKING: 5 MIN

SERVES: 1

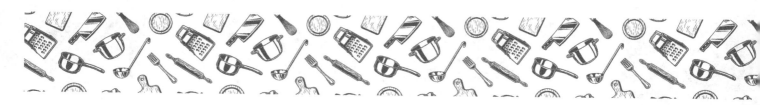

INGREDIENTS

- 3 eggs
- 1/4 cup fresh mint, chopped
- 2 tbsp coconut milk
- 1/2 tsp olive oil
- 2 tbsp feta cheese, crumbled
- Pepper
- Salt

DIRECTIONS

1. In a bowl, whisk eggs with feta cheese, mint, milk, pepper, and salt.
2. Heat olive oil in a pan over low heat. Pour egg mixture in the pan and cook until eggs are set.
3. Flip omelet and cook for 2 minutes more.
4. Serve and enjoy.

Nutritions: *Calories 275, Fat 20g, Carbohydrates 4g, Sugar 2g, Protein 20g, Cholesterol 505 mg*

31. SAUSAGE BREAKFAST CASSEROLE

PREPARATION: 10 MIN

COOKING: 50 MIN

SERVES: 8

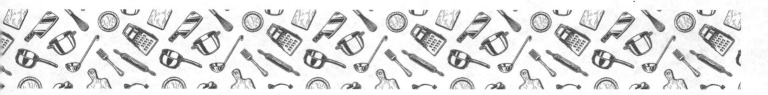

INGREDIENTS

- 12 eggs
- 1 lb. ground Italian sausage
- 2 1/2 tomatoes, sliced
- 3 tbsp coconut flour
- 1/4 cup coconut milk
- 2 small zucchinis, shredded
- Pepper
- Salt

DIRECTIONS

1. Preheat the oven to 350.
2. Spray crockpot dish with cooking spray and set aside.
3. Cook sausage in a pan until brown.
4. Transfer sausage to a mixing bowl.
5. Add coconut flour, milk, eggs, zucchini, pepper, and salt. Stir well.
6. Add eggs and whisk to combine.
7. Transfer bowl mixture into the casserole dish and top with tomato slices.
8. Bake for 50 minutes.
9. Serve and enjoy.

Nutritions: *Calories 305, Fat 21.8g, Carbohydrates 6.3g, Sugar 3.3g, Protein 19.6g, Cholesterol 286 mg*

32. MOZZARELLA CHEESE OMELET

PREPARATION: 10 MIN

COOKING: 5 MIN

SERVES: 1

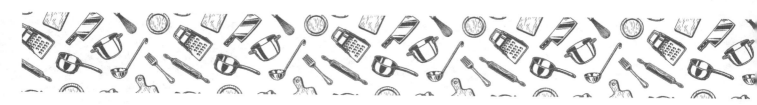

INGREDIENTS

- eggs, beaten
- 1/4 cup mozzarella cheese, shredded
- tomato slices
- 1/4 tsp Italian seasoning
- 1/4 tsp dried oregano
- Pepper
- Salt

DIRECTIONS

1. In a bowl, whisk eggs with salt.
2. Spray pan with cookery spray and heat over medium heat.
3. Pour egg mix into the pan and cook over medium heat.
4. Once eggs are set then sprinkle oregano and Italian seasoning on top.
5. Arrange tomato slices on top of the omelet and sprinkle with shredded cheese.
6. Cook omelet for 1 minute.
7. Serve and enjoy.

Nutritions: *Calories 285, Fat 19g, Carbohydrates 4g, Sugar 3g, Protein 25g, Cholesterol 655 mg*

33. CHERRY BERRY BULGUR BOWL

PREPARATION: 15 MIN

COOKING: 15 MIN

SERVES: 4

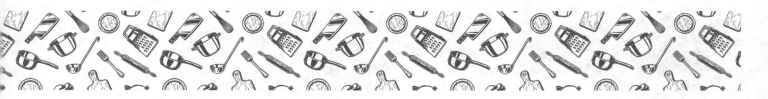

INGREDIENTS

- 1 cup medium-grind bulgur
- 2 cups water
- Pinch salt
- 1 cup halved and pitted cherries or 1 cup canned cherries, drained
- ½ cup raspberries
- ½ cup blackberries
- 1 tablespoon cherry jam
- 2 cups plain whole-milk yogurt

DIRECTIONS

1. Mix the bulgur, water, and salt in a medium saucepan. Do this in a medium heat. Bring to a boil.
2. Reduce the heat to low and simmer, partially covered, for 12 to 15 minutes or until the bulgur is almost tender. Cover, and let stand for 5 minutes to finish cooking do this after removing the pan from the heat.
3. While the bulgur is cooking, combine the raspberries and blackberries in a medium bowl. Stir the cherry jam into the fruit.
4. When the bulgur is tender, divide among four bowls. Top each bowl with ½ cup of yogurt and an equal amount of the berry mixture and serve.

Nutritions: *Calories: 242; Total fat: 6g; Saturated fat: 3g; Sodium: 85mg; Phosphorus: 237mg; Potassium: 438mg; Carbohydrates: 44g; Fiber: 7g; Protein: 9g; Sugar: 13g*

34. HEALTHY SPINACH TOMATO MUFFINS

PREPARATION: 10 MIN   **COOKING: 20 MIN**   **SERVES: 12**

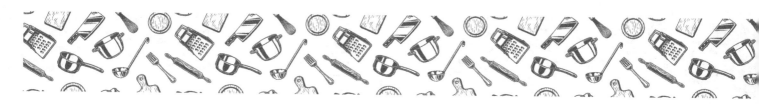

INGREDIENTS

- 12 eggs
- 1/2 tsp Italian seasoning
- 1 cup tomatoes, chopped
- tbsp water
- 1 cup fresh spinach, chopped
- Pepper
- Salt

DIRECTIONS

1. In a mixing bowl, whisk eggs with water, Italian seasoning, pepper, and salt.
2. Add spinach and tomatoes and stir well.
3. Pour egg mixture into the prepared muffin tray and bake for 20 minutes.
4. Serve and enjoy.

Nutritions: *Calories 67, Fat 4.5g, Carbohydrates 1g, Sugar 0.8g, Protein 5.7g, Cholesterol 164 mg*

35. CHICKEN EGG BREAKFAST MUFFINS

PREPARATION: 10 MIN

COOKING: 15 MIN

SERVES: 12

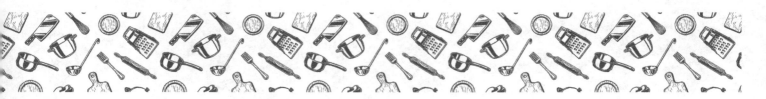

INGREDIENTS

- eggs
- 1 cup cooked chicken, chopped
- 3 tbsp green onions, chopped
- 1/4 tsp garlic powder
- Pepper
- Salt

DIRECTIONS

1. Preheat the oven to 400 F
2. Spray muffin tray with cooking spray and set aside.
3. In a big bowl, whisk eggs with garlic powder, pepper, and salt.
4. Add remaining ingredients and stir well.
5. Pour egg mixture into the muffin tray and bake for 15 minutes.
6. Serve and enjoy.

Nutritions: *Calories 71, Fat 4 g, Carbohydrates 0.4g, Sugar 0.3g, Protein 8g, Cholesterol 145 mg*

36. KETO OVERNIGHT OATS

PREPARATION: 5 MIN

COOKING: 5 MIN

SERVES: 2

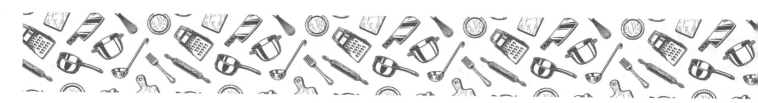

INGREDIENTS

- 1 tbsp chia seed
- drops liquid stevia
- 1/2 cup hemp hearts
- 2/3 cup coconut milk
- 1/2 tsp vanilla
- Pinch of salt

DIRECTIONS

1. Add all the ingredients into the bowl and mix well.
2. Cover and place in refrigerator for 8 hours.
3. Serve and enjoy.

Nutritions: *Calories 289, Fat 22.5g, Carbohydrates 5g, Sugar 0.1g, Protein 14g, Cholesterol 0 mg*

37. CHEESE COCONUT PANCAKES

PREPARATION: 10 MIN

COOKING: 5 MIN

SERVES: 1

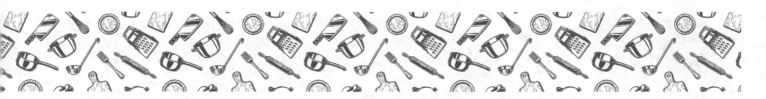

INGREDIENTS

- 2 eggs
- 1 packet stevia
- 1/2 tsp cinnamon
- 2 oz cream cheese
- 1 tbsp coconut flour
- 1/2 tsp vanilla

DIRECTIONS

1. Add all the ingredients into the bowl and blend until smooth.
2. Spray pan with cooking spray and warm over medium-high heat.
3. Pour batter on the hot pan and make two pancakes.
4. Cook pancake until lightly brown from both the sides.
5. Serve and enjoy.

Nutritions: *Calories 386, Fat 30g, Carbohydrates 12g, Sugar 1g, Protein 16g, Cholesterol 389 mg*

38. COCONUT BREAKFAST SMOOTHIE

PREPARATION: 5 MIN

COOKING: 5 MIN

SERVES: 1

INGREDIENTS

- 1/4 cup whey protein powder
- 1/2 cup coconut milk
- drops liquid stevia
- 1 tbsp coconut oil
- 1 tsp vanilla
- 2 tbsp coconut butter
- 1/4 cup water
- 1/2 cup ice

DIRECTIONS

1. Add the ingredients into the blender and blend until smooth.
2. Serve and enjoy.

Nutritions: *Calories 560, Fat 45g, Carbohydrates 12g, Sugar 4g, Protein 25g, Cholesterol 60 mg*

39. CINNAMON CHEESE PANCAKES

PREPARATION: 10 MIN

COOKING: 10 MIN

SERVES: 4

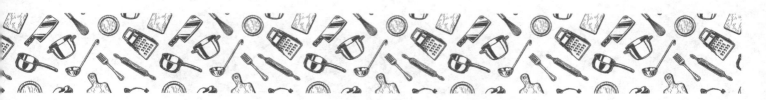

INGREDIENTS

- eggs
- 1/2 cup cream cheese
- 1/2 cup almond flour
- 1 tbsp butter, melted
- 1/2 tsp cinnamon

DIRECTIONS

1. Add all ingredients except butter into the blender and blend until well combined.
2. The heat melted butter in a pan over medium heat.
3. Pour 3 tbsp of batter on the pan and make pancakes and cook for 2 minutes on each side.
4. Serve and enjoy.

Nutritions: *Calories 271, Fat 24 g, Carbohydrates 4g, Sugar 1g, Protein 10g, Cholesterol 201 mg*

40. BREAKFAST EGG SALAD

PREPARATION: 10 MIN

COOKING: 5 MIN

SERVES: 4

INGREDIENTS

- eggs, hard-boiled, peeled and chopped
- 1/2 cup dill pickles, chopped
- 1 tbsp fresh dill, chopped
- tbsp mayonnaise

DIRECTIONS

1. Add the ingredients into the big container and stir to mix.
2. Serve and enjoy.

Nutritions: *Calories 140, Fat 10g, Carbohydrates 4g, Sugar 1g, Protein 8g, Cholesterol 245 mg*

41. CREAMY CINNAMON SCRAMBLED EGG

PREPARATION: 10 MIN

COOKING: 5 MIN

SERVES: 2

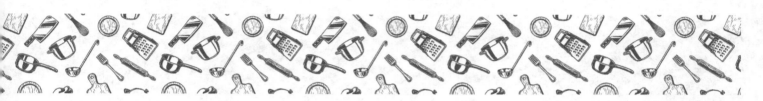

INGREDIENTS

- eggs
- 1/4 tsp ground cinnamon
- tbsp heavy cream
- 1 tbsp butter
- Pepper
- Salt

DIRECTIONS

1. In a bowl, mix together eggs and heavy cream.
2. Melt butter in a pan over medium heat.
3. Add the egg mixture in a pan and stir until eggs are cooked. Remove pan from heat.
4. Sprinkle with ground cinnamon.
5. Serve and enjoy.

Nutritions: *Calories 186, Fat 15g, Carbohydrates 1g, Sugar 1g, Protein 12g, Cholesterol 346 mg*

42. CHOCO COCONUT SMOOTHIE

PREPARATION: 5 MIN

COOKING: 5 MIN

SERVES: 1

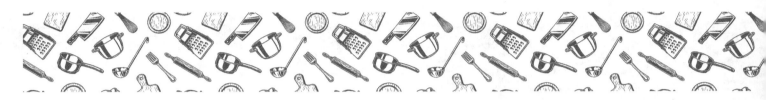

INGREDIENTS

- 1/2 tbsp cocoa powder
- 1/4 cup heavy cream
- drops liquid stevia
- 1/4 cup coconut milk
- 1/2 cup unsweetened almond milk

DIRECTIONS

1. Add the ingredients to the blender then blend until smooth.
2. Serve and enjoy.

Nutritions: *Calories 201, Fat 19g, Carbohydrates 7g, Sugar 3g, Protein 2g, Cholesterol 10 mg*

43. BERRY CHIA WITH YOGURT

PREPARATION: 35 MIN

COOKING: 5 MIN

SERVES: 4

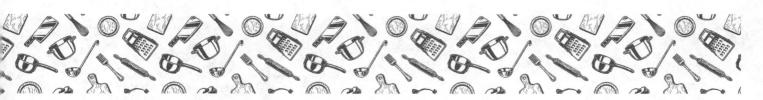

INGREDIENTS

- ½ cup chia seeds, dried
- cup Plain yogurt
- 1/3 cup strawberries, chopped
- ¼ cup blackberries
- ¼ cup raspberries
- teaspoons Splenda

DIRECTIONS

1. Mix up together Plain yogurt with Splenda, and chia seeds.
2. Transfer the mixture into the serving ramekins (jars) and leave for 35 minutes.
3. After this, add blackberries, raspberries, and strawberries. Mix up the meal well.
4. Serve it immediately or store in the fridge up to 2 days.

Nutritions: *Calories 257, Fat 10.3g, Fiber 11g, Carbs 27.2g, Protein 12g*

44. ARUGULA EGGS WITH CHILI PEPPERS

PREPARATION: 7 MIN

COOKING: 10 MIN

SERVES: 4

INGREDIENTS

- cups arugula, chopped
- eggs, beaten
- ½ chili pepper, chopped
- 1 tablespoon butter
- 1 oz Parmesan, grated

DIRECTIONS

1. Toss butter in the skillet and melt it.
2. Add arugula and sauté it over the medium heat for 5 minutes. Stir it from time to time.
3. Meanwhile, mix up together Parmesan, chili pepper, and eggs.
4. Pour the egg mixture over the arugula and scramble well.
5. Cook the breakfast for 5 minutes more over the medium heat.

Nutritions: *Calories 98, Fat 7.8g, Fiber 0.2g, Carbs 0.9g, Protein 6.7g*

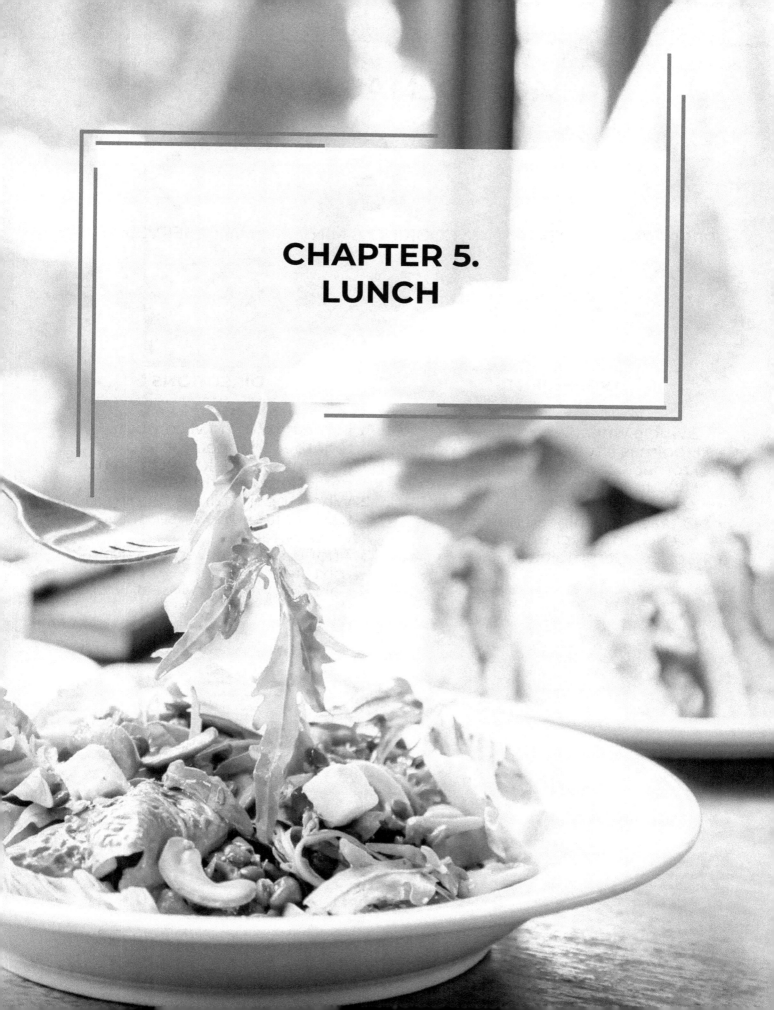

CHAPTER 5.
LUNCH

46. DOLMAS WRAP

PREPARATION: 10 MIN

COOKING: 5 MIN

SERVES: 2

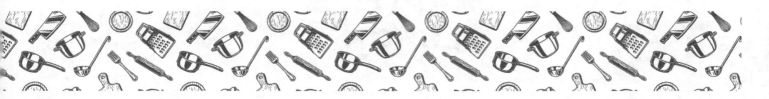

INGREDIENTS

- 2 whole wheat wraps
- 6 dolmas (stuffed grape leaves)
- 1 tomato, chopped
- 1 cucumber, chopped
- 2 oz Greek yogurt
- ½ teaspoon minced garlic
- ¼ cup lettuce, chopped
- 2 oz Feta, crumbled

DIRECTIONS

1. In the mixing bowl combine together chopped tomato, cucumber, Greek yogurt, minced garlic, lettuce, and Feta.
2. When the mixture is homogenous transfer it in the center of every wheat wrap.
3. Arrange dolma over the vegetable mixture.
4. Carefully wrap the wheat wraps.

Nutritions: *Calories 341, Fat 12.9, Fiber 9.2, Carbs 52.4, Protein 13.2*

47. SALAD AL TONNO

PREPARATION: 15 MIN

COOKING: 0 MIN

SERVES: 2

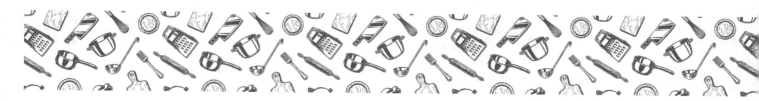

INGREDIENTS

- 1/3 cup stuffed green olives
- 1 ½ cup lettuce leaves, teared
- ½ cup cherry tomatoes, halved
- ½ teaspoon garlic powder
- ½ teaspoon salt
- ½ teaspoon ground black pepper
- 1 tablespoon lemon juice
- 1 teaspoon olive oil
- 6 oz tuna, canned, drained

DIRECTIONS

1. Chop the tuna roughly and put it in the salad bowl.
2. Add cherry tomatoes, lettuce leaves, salt, garlic powder, ground black pepper. Lemon juice, and olive oil.
3. Then slice the stuffed olives and add them in the salad too.
4. Give a good shake to the salad.

Nutritions: *Calories 235, Fat 12, Fiber 1, Carbs 6.5, Protein 23.4*

48. ARLECCHINO RICE SALAD

PREPARATION: 10 MIN

COOKING: 15 MIN

SERVES: 3

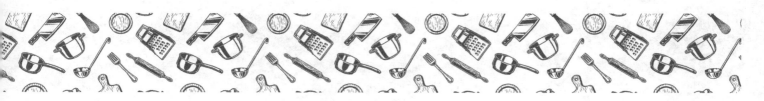

INGREDIENTS

- ½ cup white rice, dried
- 1 cup chicken stock
- 1 zucchini, shredded
- 2 tablespoons capers
- 1 carrot, shredded
- 1 tomato, chopped
- 1 tablespoon apple cider vinegar
- ½ teaspoon salt
- 2 tablespoons fresh parsley, chopped
- 1 tablespoon canola oil

DIRECTIONS

1. Put rice in the pan.
2. Add chicken stock and boil it with the closed lid for 15-20 minutes or until rice absorbs all water.
3. Meanwhile, in the mixing bowl combine together shredded zucchini, capers, carrot, and tomato.
4. Add fresh parsley.
5. Make the dressing: mix up together canola oil, salt, and apple cider vinegar.
6. Chill the cooked rice little and add it in the salad bowl to the vegetables.
7. Add dressing and mix up salad well.

Nutritions: *Calories 183, Fat 5.3, Fiber 2.1, Carbs 30.4, Protein 3.8*

49. GREEK SALAD

PREPARATION: 10 MIN

COOKING: 0 MIN

SERVES: 2

INGREDIENTS

- 2 cups lettuce leaves
- 4 oz black olives
- 2 tomatoes
- 2 cucumbers
- 1 tablespoon lemon juice
- 1 teaspoon olive oil
- ¼ teaspoon dried oregano
- ½ teaspoon salt
- ¼ teaspoon chili flakes
- 4 oz Feta cheese

DIRECTIONS

1. Chop Feta cheese into the small cubes.
2. Chop the lettuce leaves roughly put them in the salad bowl.
3. Slice black olives and add them in the lettuce.
4. Then chop tomatoes and cucumbers into the cubes. Add them in the lettuce bowl.
5. For the dressing: whisk together chili flakes, salt, dried oregano, olive oil, and lemon juice.
6. Pour the dressing over the lettuce mixture and mix up well.
7. Sprinkle the salad with Feta cubes and shake gently.

Nutritions: *Calories 312, Fat 21.2, Fiber 5.3, Carbs 23.5, Protein 11.9*

50. SAUTEED CHICKPEA AND LENTIL MIX

PREPARATION: 10 MIN

COOKING: 50 MIN

SERVES: 4

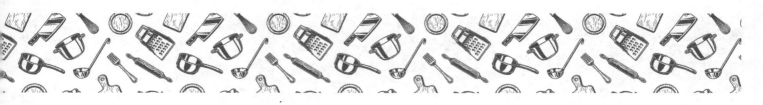

INGREDIENTS

- 1 cup chickpeas, half-cooked
- 1 cup lentils
- 5 cups chicken stock
- ½ cup fresh cilantro, chopped
- 1 teaspoon salt
- ½ teaspoon chili flakes
- ¼ cup onion, diced
- 1 tablespoon tomato paste

DIRECTIONS

1. Place chickpeas in the pan.
2. Add water, salt, and chili flakes.
3. Boil the chickpeas for 30 minutes over the medium heat.
4. Then add diced onion, lentils, and tomato paste. Stir well.
5. Close the lid and cook the mix for 15 minutes.
6. After this, add chopped cilantro, stir the meal well and cook it for 5 minutes more.
7. Let the cooked lunch chill little before serving.

Nutritions: *Calories 370, Fat 4.3, Fiber 23.7, Carbs 61.6, Protein 23.2*

51. BUFFALO CHICKEN LETTUCE WRAPS

PREPARATION: 35 MIN

COOKING: 10 MIN

SERVES: 2

INGREDIENTS

- 3 chicken breasts, boneless and cubed
- 20 slices of almond butter lettuce leaves
- ¾ cup cherry tomatoes halved
- 1 avocado, chopped
- ¼ cup green onions, diced
- ½ cup ranch dressing
- ¾ cup hot sauce

DIRECTIONS

1. Take a mixing bowl and add chicken cubes and hot sauce, mix.
2. Place in the fridge and let it marinate for 30 minutes.
3. Preheat your oven to 400 degrees F.
4. Place coated chicken on a cookie pan and bake for 9 minutes.
5. Assemble lettuce serving cups with equal amounts of lettuce, green onions, tomatoes, ranch dressing, and cubed chicken.
6. Serve and enjoy!

Nutritions: *Calories: 106, Fat: 6g Net, Carbohydrates: 2g, Protein: 5g*

52. CRAZY JAPANESE POTATO AND BEEF CROQUETTES

PREPARATION: 10 MIN

COOKING: 20 MIN

SERVES: 10

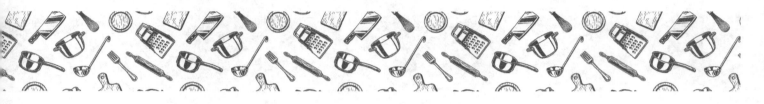

INGREDIENTS

- 3 medium russet potatoes, peeled and chopped
- 1 tablespoon almond butter
- 1 tablespoon vegetable oil
- 3 onions, diced
- ¾ pound ground beef
- 4 teaspoons light coconut aminos
- All-purpose flour for coating
- 2 eggs, beaten
- Panko bread crumbs for coating
- ½ cup oil, frying

DIRECTIONS

1. Take a saucepan and place it over medium-high heat; add potatoes and sunflower seeds water, boil for 16 minutes.
2. Remove water and put potatoes in another bowl, add almond butter and mash the potatoes.
3. Take a frying pan and place it over medium heat, add 1 tablespoon oil and let it heat up.
4. Add onions and stir fry until tender.
5. Add coconut aminos to beef to onions.
6. Keep frying until beef is browned.
7. Mix the beef with the potatoes evenly.
8. Take another frying pan and place it over medium heat; add half a cup of oil.
9. Form croquettes using the mashed potato mixture and coat them with flour, then eggs and finally breadcrumbs.
10. Fry patties until golden on all sides.
11. Enjoy!

Nutritions: *Calories: 239 Fat: 4g Carbohydrates: 20g Protein: 10g*

53. SPICY CHILI CRACKERS

PREPARATION: 15 MIN

COOKING: 60 MIN

SERVES: 30 CRACKERS

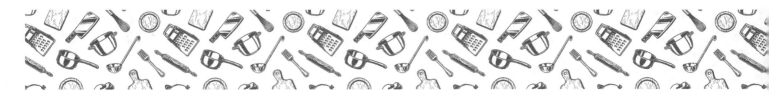

INGREDIENTS

- ¾ cup almond flour
- ¼ cup coconut four
- ¼ cup coconut flour
- ½ teaspoon paprika
- ½ teaspoon cumin
- 1 ½ teaspoons chili pepper spice
- 1 teaspoon onion powder
- ½ teaspoon sunflower seeds
- 1 whole egg
- ¼ cup unsalted almond butter

DIRECTIONS

1. Preheat your oven to 350 degrees F.
2. Add ingredients to your food processor and pulse until you have a nice dough.
3. Divide dough into two equal parts.
4. Place one ball on a sheet of parchment paper and cover with another sheet; roll it out.
5. Cut into crackers and repeat with the other ball.
6. Transfer the prepped dough to a baking tray and bake for 8-10 minutes.
7. Remove from oven and serve.
8. Enjoy!

Nutritions: *Total Carbs: 2.8g, Fiber: 1g, Protein: 1.6g, Fat: 4.1g*

54. GOLDEN EGGPLANT FRIES

PREPARATION: 10 MIN

COOKING: 15 MIN

SERVES: 8

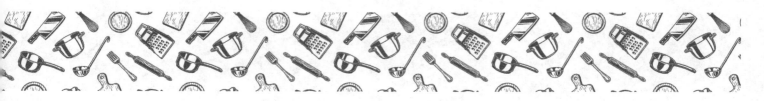

INGREDIENTS

- 2 eggs
- 2 cups almond flour
- 2 tablespoons coconut oil, spray
- 2 eggplant, peeled and cut thinly
- Sunflower seeds and pepper

DIRECTIONS

1. Preheat your oven to 400 degrees F.
2. Take a bowl and mix with sunflower seeds and black pepper.
3. Take another bowl and beat eggs until frothy.
4. Dip the eggplant pieces into the eggs.
5. Then coat them with the flour mixture.
6. Add another layer of flour and egg.
7. Then, take a baking sheet and grease with coconut oil on top.
8. Bake for about 15 minutes.
9. Serve and enjoy!

Nutritions: *Calories: 212, Fat: 15.8g, Carbohydrates: 12.1g, Protein: 8.6g*

55. TRADITIONAL BLACK BEAN CHILI

PREPARATION: 10 MIN

COOKING: 4 H

SERVES: 4

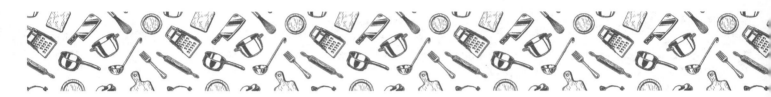

INGREDIENTS

- 1 ½ cups red bell pepper, chopped
- 1 cup yellow onion, chopped
- 1 ½ cups mushrooms, sliced
- 1 tablespoon olive oil
- 1 tablespoon chili powder
- 2 garlic cloves, minced
- 1 teaspoon chipotle chili pepper, chopped
- ½ teaspoon cumin, ground
- 2 tablespoons cilantro, chopped
- 1 cup tomatoes, chopped

DIRECTIONS

1. Add red bell peppers, onion, dill, mushrooms, chili powder, garlic, chili pepper, cumin, black beans, tomatoes to your Slow Cooker.
2. Stir well.
3. Place lid and cook on HIGH for 4 hours.
4. Sprinkle cilantro on top.
5. Serve and enjoy!

Nutritions: *Calories: 211, Fat: 3g, Carbohydrates: 22g, Protein: 5g*

56. VERY WILD MUSHROOM PILAF

PREPARATION: 10 MIN

COOKING: 3 H

SERVES: 4

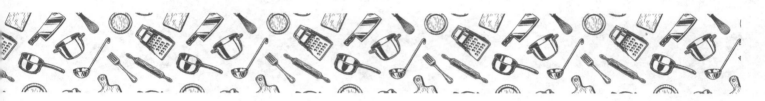

INGREDIENTS

- 1 cup wild rice
- 2 garlic cloves, minced
- 6 green onions, chopped
- 2 tablespoons olive oil
- ½ pound baby Bella mushrooms
- 2 cups water

DIRECTIONS

1. Add rice, garlic, onion, oil, mushrooms and water to your Slow Cooker.
2. Stir well until mixed.
3. Place the lid and cook on LOW for 3 hours.
4. Stir pilaf and divide between serving platters.
5. Enjoy!

Nutritions: *Calories: 210 Fat: 7g Carbohydrates: 16g Protein: 4g*

57. GREEN PALAK PANEER

PREPARATION: 5 MIN

COOKING: 10 MIN

SERVES: 4

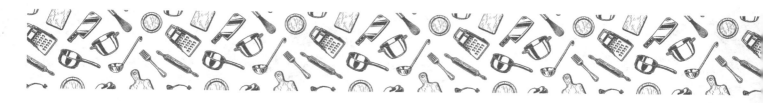

INGREDIENTS

- 1-pound spinach
- 2 cups cubed paneer (vegan)
- 2 tablespoons coconut oil
- 1 teaspoon cumin
- 1 chopped up onion
- 1-2 teaspoons hot green chili minced up
- 1 teaspoon minced garlic
- 15 cashews
- 4 tablespoons almond milk
- 1 teaspoon Garam masala
- Flavored vinegar as needed

DIRECTIONS

1. Add cashews and milk to a blender and blend well.
2. Set your pot to Sauté mode and add coconut oil; allow the oil to heat up.
3. Add cumin seeds, garlic, green chilies, ginger and sauté for 1 minute.
4. Add onion and sauté for 2 minutes.
5. Add chopped spinach, flavored vinegar and a cup of water.
6. Lock up the lid and cook on HIGH pressure for 10 minutes.
7. Quick-release the pressure.
8. Add ½ cup of water and blend to a paste.
9. Add cashew paste, paneer and Garam Masala and stir thoroughly.
10. Serve over hot rice!

Nutritions: *Calories:367, Fat: 26g, Carbohydrates: 21g, Protein: 16g*

58. SPORTY BABY CARROTS

PREPARATION: 5 MIN

COOKING: 5 MIN

SERVES: 4

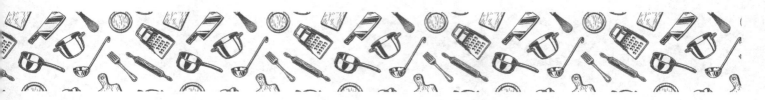

INGREDIENTS

- 1-pound baby carrots
- 1 cup water
- 1 tablespoon clarified ghee
- 1 tablespoon chopped up fresh mint leaves
- Sea flavored vinegar as needed

DIRECTIONS

1. Place steamer rack on top of your pot and add the carrots.
2. Add water.
3. Lock the lid and cook at HIGH pressure for 2 minutes.
4. Do a quick release.
5. Pass the carrots through a strainer and drain them.
6. Wipe the insert clean.
7. Return insert to the pot and set the pot to Sauté mode.
8. Add clarified butter and allow it to melt.
9. Add mint and sauté for 30 seconds.
10. Add carrots to the insert and sauté well.
11. Remove them and sprinkle with bit of flavored vinegar on top.
12. Enjoy!

Nutritions: *Calories:131, Fat: 10g, Carbohydrates: 11g, Protein: 1g*

59. SAUCY GARLIC GREENS

PREPARATION: 5 MIN

COOKING: 20 MIN

SERVES: 4

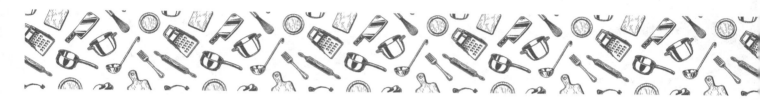

INGREDIENTS

- 1 bunch of leafy greens
- Sauce
- ½ cup cashews soaked in water for 10 minutes
- ¼ cup water
- 1 tablespoon lemon juice
- 1 teaspoon coconut aminos
- 1 clove peeled whole clove
- 1/8 teaspoon of flavored vinegar

DIRECTIONS

1. Make the sauce by draining and discarding the soaking water from your cashews and add the cashews to a blender.
2. Add fresh water, lemon juice, flavored vinegar, coconut aminos, garlic.
3. Blitz until you have a smooth cream and transfer to bowl.
4. Add ½ cup of water to the pot.
5. Place the steamer basket to the pot and add the greens in the basket.
6. Lock the lid and steam for 1 minute.
7. Quick-release the pressure.
8. Transfer the steamed greens to strainer and extract excess water.
9. Place the greens into a mixing bowl.
10. Add lemon garlic sauce and toss.
11. Enjoy!

Nutritions: *Calories:77, Fat: 5g, Carbohydrates: 0g, Protein: 2g*

60. GARDEN SALAD

PREPARATION: 5 MIN

COOKING: 20 MIN

SERVES: 6

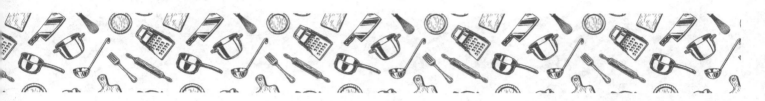

INGREDIENTS

- 1-pound raw peanuts in shell
- 1 bay leaf
- 2 medium-sized chopped up tomatoes
- ½ cup diced up green pepper
- ½ cup diced up sweet onion
- ¼ cup finely diced hot pepper
- ¼ cup diced up celery
- 2 tablespoons olive oil
- ¾ teaspoon flavored vinegar
- ¼ teaspoon freshly ground black pepper

DIRECTIONS

1. Boil your peanuts for 1 minute and rinse them.
2. The skin will be soft, so discard the skin.
3. Add 2 cups of water to the Instant Pot.
4. Add bay leaf and peanuts.
5. Lock the lid and cook on HIGH pressure for 20 minutes.
6. Drain the water.
7. Take a large bowl and add the peanuts, diced up vegetables.
8. Whisk in olive oil, lemon juice, pepper in another bowl.
9. Pour the mixture over the salad and mix.
10. Enjoy!

Nutritions: *Calories:140, Fat: 4g, Carbohydrates: 24g, Protein: 5g*

61. SPICY CABBAGE DISH

PREPARATION: 10 MIN

COOKING: 4 H

SERVES: 4

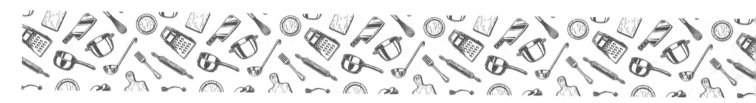

INGREDIENTS

- 2 yellow onions, chopped
- 10 cups red cabbage, shredded
- 1 cup plums, pitted and chopped
- 1 teaspoon cinnamon powder
- 1 garlic clove, minced
- 1 teaspoon cumin seeds
- ¼ teaspoon cloves, ground
- 2 tablespoons red wine vinegar
- 1 teaspoon coriander seeds
- ½ cup water

DIRECTIONS

1. Add cabbage, onion, plums, garlic, cumin, cinnamon, cloves, vinegar, coriander and water to your Slow Cooker.
2. Stir well.
3. Place lid and cook on LOW for 4 hours.
4. Divide between serving platters.
5. Enjoy!

Nutritions: *Calories: 197, Fat: 1g, Carbohydrates: 14g, Protein: 3g*

62. EXTREME BALSAMIC CHICKEN

PREPARATION: 10 MIN

COOKING: 35 MIN

SERVES: 4

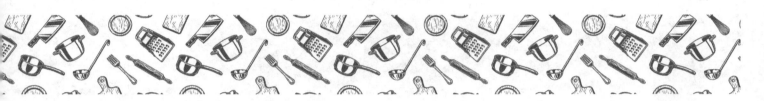

INGREDIENTS

- 3 boneless chicken breasts, skinless
- Sunflower seeds to taste
- ¼ cup almond flour
- 2/3 cups low-fat chicken broth
- 1 ½ teaspoons arrowroot
- ½ cup low sugar raspberry preserve
- 1 ½ tablespoons balsamic vinegar

DIRECTIONS

1. Dredge the chicken pieces in flour and shake off any excess.
2. Take a non-stick skillet and place it over medium heat.
3. Add chicken to the skillet and cook for 15 minutes, making sure to turn them half-way through.
4. Remove chicken and transfer to platter.
5. Add arrowroot, broth, raspberry preserve to the skillet and stir.
6. Stir in balsamic vinegar and reduce heat to low, stir-cook for a few minutes.
7. Transfer the chicken back to the sauce and cook for 15 minutes more.
8. Serve and enjoy!

Nutritions: *Calories: 546, Fat: 35g, Carbohydrates: 11g, Protein: 44g*

63. ENJOYABLE SPINACH AND BEAN MEDLEY

PREPARATION: 10 MIN

COOKING: 4 H

SERVES: 4

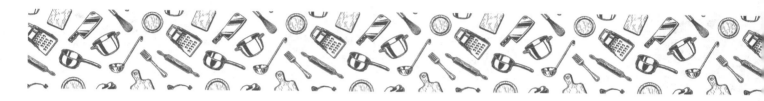

INGREDIENTS

- 5 carrots, sliced
- 1 ½ cups great northern beans, dried
- 2 garlic cloves, minced
- 1 yellow onion, chopped
- Pepper to taste
- ½ teaspoon oregano, dried
- 5 ounces baby spinach
- 4 ½ cups low sodium veggie stock
- 2 teaspoons lemon peel, grated
- 3 tablespoon lemon juice

DIRECTIONS

1. Add beans, onion, carrots, garlic, oregano and stock to your Slow Cooker.
2. Stir well.
3. Place lid and cook on HIGH for 4 hours.
4. Add spinach, lemon juice and lemon peel.
5. Stir and let it sit for 5 minutes.
6. Divide between serving platters and enjoy!

Nutritions: *Calories: 219, Fat: 8g, Carbohydrates: 14g, Protein: 8g*

64. TANTALIZING CAULIFLOWER AND DILL MASH

PREPARATION: 10 MIN

COOKING: 6 H

SERVES: 6

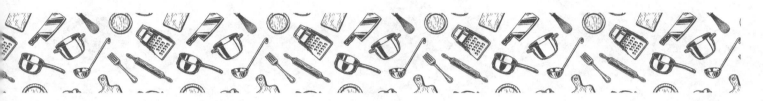

INGREDIENTS

- 1 cauliflower head, florets separated
- 1/3 cup dill, chopped
- 6 garlic cloves
- 2 tablespoons olive oil
- Pinch of black pepper

DIRECTIONS

1. Add cauliflower to Slow Cooker.
2. Add dill, garlic and water to cover them.
3. Place lid and cook on HIGH for 5 hours.
4. Drain the flowers.
5. Season with pepper and add oil, mash using potato masher.
6. Whisk and serve.
7. Enjoy!

Nutritions: *Calories: 207, Fat: 4g, Carbohydrates: 14g, Protein: 3g*

65. SECRET ASIAN GREEN BEANS

PREPARATION: 10 MIN

COOKING: 2 H

SERVES: 10

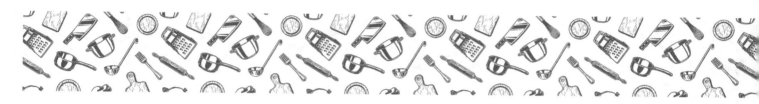

INGREDIENTS

- 16 cups green beans, halved
- 3 tablespoons olive oil
- ¼ cup tomato sauce, salt-free
- ½ cup coconut sugar
- ¾ teaspoon low sodium soy sauce
- Pinch of pepper

DIRECTIONS

1. Add green beans, coconut sugar, pepper tomato sauce, soy sauce, oil to your Slow Cooker.
2. Stir well.
3. Place the lid and cook on LOW for 3 hours.
4. Divide between serving platters and serve.
5. Enjoy!

Nutritions: *Calories: 200, Fat: 4g, Carbohydrates: 12g, Protein: 3g*

66. EXCELLENT ACORN MIX

PREPARATION: 10 MIN   **COOKING: 7 H**   **SERVES: 10**

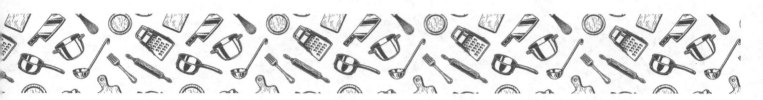

INGREDIENTS

- 2 acorn squash, peeled and cut into wedges
- 16 ounces cranberry sauce, unsweetened
- ¼ teaspoon cinnamon powder
- Pepper to taste

DIRECTIONS

1. Add acorn wedges to your Slow Cooker.
2. Add cranberry sauce, cinnamon, raisins and pepper.
3. Stir.
4. Place lid and cook on LOW for 7 hours.
5. Serve and enjoy!

Nutritions: *Calories: 200, Fat: 3g, Carbohydrates: 15g, Protein: 2g*

67. BEEF CHIMICHANGAS

PREPARATION: 10 MIN

COOKING: 10-12 H

SERVES: 16

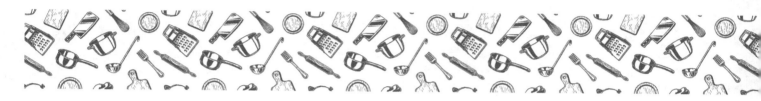

INGREDIENTS

- Shredded beef
- 3lb boneless beef chuck roast, fat trimmed away
- 3 tablespoon low-sodium taco seasoning mix
- 1 10ounce canned low-sodium diced tomatoes
- 6ounce canned diced green chilies with the juice
- 3 garlic cloves, minced
- To serve
- 16 medium flour tortillas
- Sodium-free refried beans
- Mexican rice, sour cream, cheddar cheese
- Guacamole, salsa, lettuce

DIRECTIONS

1. Arrange the beef in a 5-quart or larger slow cooker.
2. Sprinkle over taco seasoning and coat well.
3. Add tomatoes and garlic and cover.
4. Cook on low for 10 to 12 hours.
5. When cooked remove the beef and shred.
6. Make burritos out of the shredded beef, refried beans, mexican rice, and cheese.
7. Bake for 10 minutes at 350° until brown.
8. Serve with salsa, lettuce, and guacamole.

Nutritions: *Calories 249, Fat 18g, Carbs 3g, Protein 33g, Fiber 5g, Potassium 633mg, Sodium 457mg*

68. MEAT LOAF

PREPARATION: 5 MIN

COOKING: 5-6 H

SERVES: 6

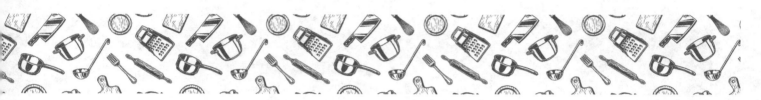

INGREDIENTS

- 2-pound lean ground beef
- 2 whole eggs, beaten
- ¾ cup milk
- ¾ cup breadcrumbs
- ½ cup chicken broth (see recipe)
- ¼ cup onion, finely diced
- 3 garlic cloves, minced
- 1 teaspoon low-sodium salt
- ¼ teaspoon freshly ground black pepper
- ¼ cup low sodium chili sauce
- Nonstick spray

DIRECTIONS

1. Mix the beaten eggs, milk, oatmeal, spices, onion, garlic, and chicken broth until well combined.
2. Mix in the beef and place in a 5-quart or larger slow cooker, sprayed with nonstick spray.
3. Cover & cook on low for 5 to 6 hours.
4. Serve with low-sodium ketchup.

Nutritions: *Calories 280, Fat 10g, Carbs 9g, Protein 37g, Fiber 1g, Potassium 648mg, Sodium 325mg*

69. CROCKPOT PEACHY PORK CHOPS

PREPARATION: 30 MIN

COOKING: 2-3 H

SERVES: 8

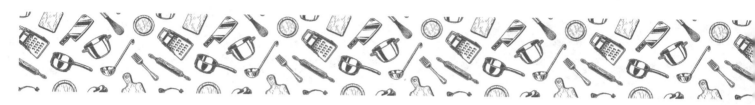

INGREDIENTS

- 4 large peaches, pitted and peeled
- 1 onion, finely minced
- ¼ cup ketchup
- ¼ cup low-sodium honey barbecue sauce
- 2 tablespoon brown sugar
- 1 tablespoon low sodium soy sauce
- ¼ teaspoon low-sodium garlic salt
- ½ teaspoon ground ginger
- 2lb boneless pork chops
- 3 tablespoon olive oil

DIRECTIONS

1. Puree the peaches with a blender.
2. Mix the peach puree with the onion, ketchup, barbecue sauce, brown sugar, soy sauce, salt, garlic salt, and ginger.
3. Brown the pork chops in a large skillet then transfer to a 6-quart or larger slow cooker.
4. Pour the sauce over the pork chops and cover.
5. Cook for 5 to 6 hours on high.

Nutritions: *Calories 252, Fat 8g, Carbs 18g, Protein 26g, Fiber 1g, Potassium 710mg, Sodium 325mg*

70. BREAKFAST SKILLET

PREPARATION: 7 MIN **COOKING: 25 MIN** **SERVES: 5**

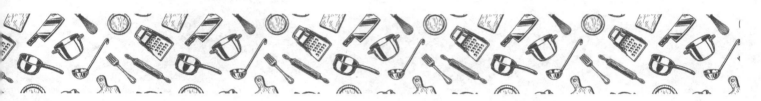

INGREDIENTS

- 1 cup cauliflower, chopped
- 1 tablespoon olive oil
- ½ red onion, diced
- 1 tablespoon Plain yogurt
- ½ teaspoon ground black pepper
- 1 teaspoon dried cilantro
- 1 teaspoon dried oregano
- 1 bell pepper, chopped
- 1/3 cup milk
- ½ teaspoon Za'atar
- 1 tablespoon lemon juice
- 1 russet potato, chopped

DIRECTIONS

1. Pour olive oil in the skillet and preheat it.
2. Add chopped russet potato and roast it for 5 minutes.
3. After this, add cauliflower, ground black pepper, cilantro, oregano, and bell pepper.
4. Roast the mixture for 10 minutes over the medium heat.
5. Then add milk, Za'atar, and Plain Yogurt. Stir it well.
6. Sauté the mixture 10 minutes
7. Top the cooked meal with diced red onion and sprinkle with lemon juice.
8. It is recommended to serve the breakfast hot.

Nutritions: *Calories 112, Fat 3.4g, Fiber 2.6g, Carbs 18.1g, Protein 3.1g*

71. PEANUT BUTTER BREAD PUDDING CUPS

PREPARATION: 10 MIN | COOKING: 20 MIN | SERVES: 6

INGREDIENTS

- Baking spray
- 5 slices whole-wheat bread, coarsely crumbled
- 2 large eggs
- ½ cup unsweetened almond milk
- ¼ cup peanut butter
- 2 tablespoons honey
- 1 teaspoon vanilla
- ½ cup chopped unsalted peanuts

DIRECTIONS

1. Preheat the oven to 375°f. And then spray a 6-cup muffin tin with baking spray and set aside.
2. Put the breadcrumbs in a medium bowl.
3. Beat the eggs, milk, peanut butter, honey, and vanilla until smooth. Pour over the breadcrumbs.
4. Stir gently until combined, then divide the mixture evenly among the muffin cups. Sprinkle with the peanuts.
5. Bake this for 18-20 minutes or until the puddings are set. Serve warm.

Nutritions: *Calories: 261; Total Fat: 15g; Saturated Fat: 3g; Sodium: 220mg; Phosphorus: 176mg; Potassium: 261mg; Carbohydrates: 24g; Fiber: 3g; Protein: 12g; Sugar: 9g*

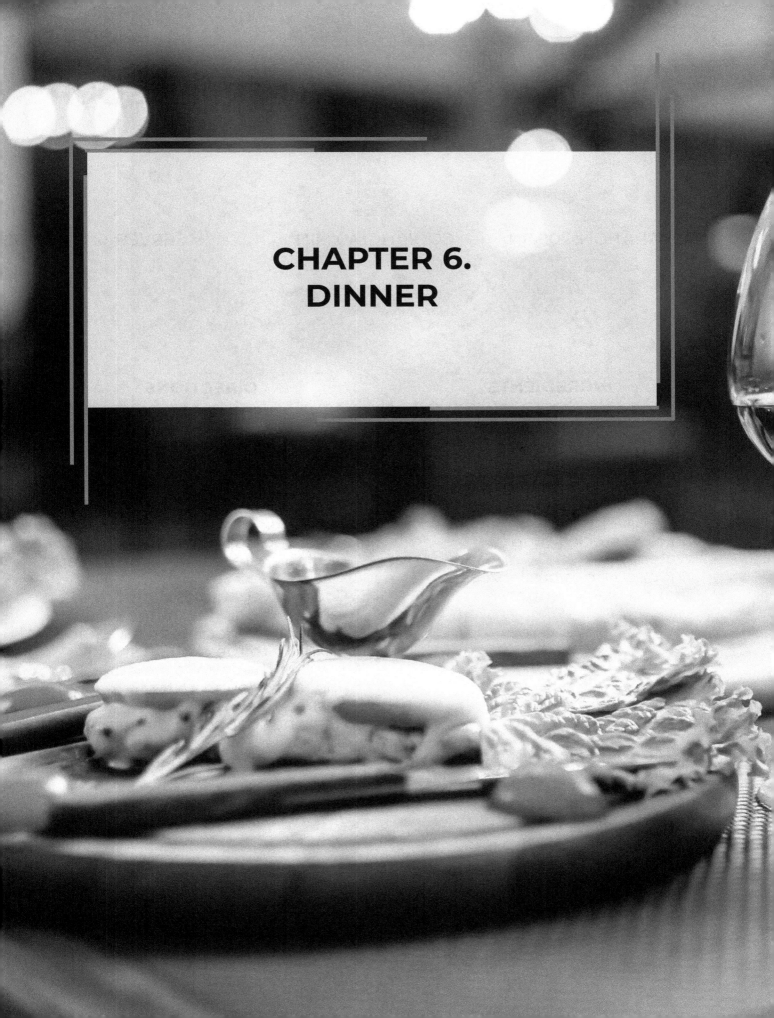

CHAPTER 6.
DINNER

72. EGGPLANT AND RED PEPPER SOUP

PREPARATION: 20 MIN

COOKING: 40 MIN

SERVES: 6

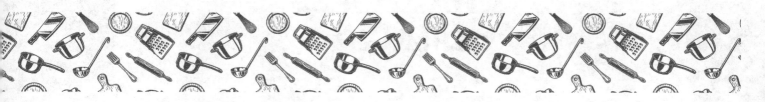

INGREDIENTS

- Sweet onion – 1 small, cut into quarters
- Small red bell peppers – 2, halved
- Cubed eggplant – 2 cups
- Garlic – 2 cloves, crushed
- Olive oil – 1 Tbsp.
- Chicken stock – 1 cup
- Water
- Chopped fresh basil – ¼ cup
- Ground black pepper

DIRECTIONS

1. Preheat the oven to 350F.
2. Put the onions, red peppers, eggplant, and garlic in a baking dish.
3. Drizzle the vegetables with the olive oil.
4. Roast vegetables for 30 minutes or until they are slightly charred and soft.
5. Cool the vegetables slightly and remove the skin from the peppers.
6. Puree the vegetables with a hand mixer (with the chicken stock).
7. Transfer the soup to a medium pot and add enough water to reach the desired thickness.
8. Heat the soup to a simmer and add the basil.
9. Season with pepper and serve.

Nutritions: *Calories: 61, Fat: 2g, Carb: 9g, Phosphorus: 33mg, Potassium: 198mg, Sodium: 98mg, Protein: 2g*

73. SEAFOOD CASSEROLE

PREPARATION: 20 MIN

COOKING: 45 MIN

SERVES: 6

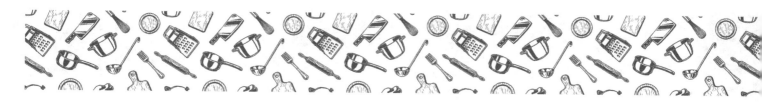

INGREDIENTS

- Eggplant – 2 cups, peeled and diced into 1-inch pieces
- Butter, for greasing the baking dish
- Olive oil – 1 tbsp.
- Sweet onion – ½, chopped
- Minced garlic - 1 tsp.
- Celery stalk – 1, chopped
- Red bell pepper – ½, boiled and chopped
- Freshly squeezed lemon juice - 3 Tbsps.
- Hot sauce – 1 tsp.
- Creole seasoning mix – ¼ tsp.
- White rice – ½ cup, uncooked
- Egg – 1 large
- Cooked shrimp – 4 ounces
- Queen crab meat – 6 ounces

DIRECTIONS

1. Preheat the oven to 350F.
2. Boil the eggplant in a saucepan for 5 minutes. Drain and set aside.
3. Grease a 9-by-13-inch baking dish with butter and set aside.
4. Heat olive oil in a large skillet over medium heat.
5. Sauté the garlic, onion, celery, and bell pepper for 4 minutes or until tender.
6. Add the sautéed vegetables to the eggplant, along with the lemon juice, hot sauce, seasoning, rice, and egg.
7. Stir to combine.
8. Fold in the shrimp and crab meat.
9. Spoon the casserole mixture into the casserole dish, patting down the top.
10. Bake for 25 to 30 minutes or until casserole is heated through and rice is tender.
11. Serve warm.

Nutritions: *Calories: 118, Fat: 4g, Carb: 9g, Phosphorus: 102mg, Potassium: 199mg, Sodium: 235mg, Protein: 12g*

74. GROUND BEEF AND RICE SOUP

PREPARATION: 15 MIN

COOKING: 40 MIN

SERVES: 6

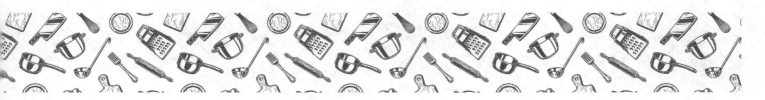

INGREDIENTS

- Extra-lean ground beef – ½ pound
- Small sweet onion – ½, chopped
- Minced garlic – 1 tsp.
- Water – 2 cups
- Low-sodium beef broth – 1 cup
- Long-grain white rice – ½ cup, uncooked
- Celery stalk – 1, chopped
- Fresh green beans – ½ cup, cut into – 1-inch pieces
- Chopped fresh thyme – 1 tsp.
- Ground black pepper

DIRECTIONS

1. Sauté the ground beef in a saucepan for 6 minutes or until the beef is completely browned.
2. Drain off the excess fat and add the onion and garlic to the saucepan.
3. Sauté the vegetables for about 3 minutes, or until they are softened.
4. Add the celery, rice, beef broth, and water.
5. Bring soup to a boil, reduce the heat to low and simmer for 30 minutes or until the rice is tender.
6. Add the green beans and thyme and simmer for 3 minutes.
7. Remove soup from the heat and season with pepper.

Nutritions: *Calories: 154, Fat: 7g, Carb: 14g, Phosphorus: 76mg, Potassium: 179mg, Sodium: 133mg, Protein: 9g*

75. COUSCOUS BURGERS

PREPARATION: 20 MIN

COOKING: 10 MIN

SERVES: 4

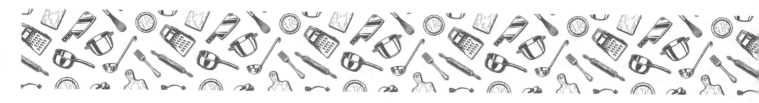

INGREDIENTS

- Canned chickpeas – ½ cup, rinsed and drained
- Chopped fresh cilantro – 2 Tbsps.
- Chopped fresh parsley
- Lemon juice - 1 Tbsp.
- Lemon zest – 2 tsps.
- Minced garlic – 1 tsp.
- Cooked couscous – 2 ½ cups
- Eggs – 2 lightly beaten
- Olive oil – 2 Tbsps.

DIRECTIONS

1. Put the cilantro, chickpeas, parsley, lemon juice, lemon zest, and garlic in a food processor and pulse until a paste form.
2. Transfer chickpea mixture to a bowl and add the eggs and couscous. Mix well.
3. Chill the mixture in the refrigerator for 1 hour.
4. Form the couscous mixture into 4 patties.
5. Heat olive oil in a skillet.
6. Place the patties in the skillet, 2 at a time, gently pressing them down with a spatula.
7. Cook for 5 min or until golden and flip the patties over.
8. Cook the other side for 5 minutes and transfer the cooked burgers to a plate covered with a paper towel.
9. Repeat with the remaining 2 burgers.

Nutritions: *Calories: 242, Fat: 10g, Carb: 29g, Phosphorus: 108mg, Potassium: 168mg, Sodium: 43mg, Protein: 9g*

76. BAKED FLOUNDER

PREPARATION: 20 MIN **COOKING: 5 MIN** **SERVES: 4**

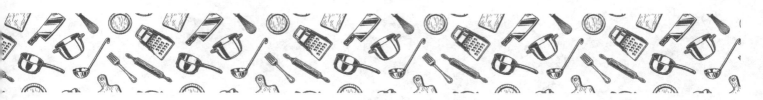

INGREDIENTS

- Homemade mayonnaise – ¼ cup
- Juice of 1 lime
- Zest of 1 lime
- Chopped fresh cilantro – ½ cup
- Flounder fillets – 4 (3-ounce)
- Ground black pepper

DIRECTIONS

1. Preheat the oven to 400F.
2. In a bowl, stir together the cilantro, lime juice, lime zest, and mayonnaise.
3. Place 4 pieces of foil, about 8 by 8 inches square, on a clean work surface.
4. Place a flounder fillet in the center of each square.
5. Top the fillets evenly with the mayonnaise mixture.
6. Season the flounder with pepper.
7. Fold sides of the foil over the fish, creating a snug packet, and place the foil packets on a baking sheet.
8. Bake the fish for 4 to 5 minutes.
9. Unfold the packets and serve.

Nutritions: *Calories: 92, Fat: 4g, Carb: 2g, Phosphorus: 208mg, Potassium: 137mg, Sodium: 267mg, Protein: 12g*

77. PERSIAN CHICKEN

PREPARATION: 10 MIN

COOKING: 20 MIN

SERVES: 5

INGREDIENTS

- Sweet onion – ½, chopped
- Lemon juice – ¼ cup
- Dried oregano – 1 Tbsp.
- Minced garlic – 1 tsp.
- Sweet paprika – 1 tsp.
- Ground cumin – ½ tsp.
- Olive oil – ½ cup
- Boneless, skinless chicken thighs – 5

DIRECTIONS

1. Put the cumin, paprika, garlic, oregano, lemon juice, and onion in a food processor and pulse to mix the ingredients.
2. Keep motor running and add the olive oil until the mixture is smooth.
3. Place chicken thighs in a large sealable freezer bag and pour the marinade into the bag.
4. Seal the bag and place in the refrigerator, turning the bag twice, for 2 hours.
5. Remove thighs from the marinade and discard the extra marinade.
6. Preheat the barbecue to medium.
7. Grill chicken for about 20 minutes, turning once, until it reaches 165F.

Nutritions: *Calories: 321, Fat: 21g, Carb: 3g, Phosphorus: 131mg, Potassium: 220mg, Sodium: 86mg, Protein: 22g*

78. SUN-DRIED TOMATO FRITTATA

PREPARATION: 10 MIN

COOKING: 20 MIN

SERVES: 8

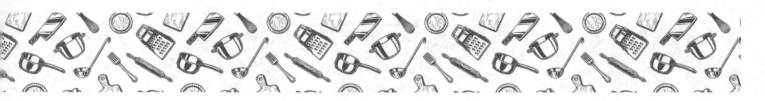

INGREDIENTS

- 12 eggs
- 1/2 tsp dried basil
- 1/4 cup parmesan cheese, grated
- cups baby spinach, shredded
- 1/4 cup sun-dried tomatoes, sliced
- Pepper
- Salt

DIRECTIONS

1. Preheat oven to 425 F. In a large bowl, whisk eggs with pepper and salt.
2. Add remaining ingredients and stir to combine.
3. Spray oven-safe pan with cooking spray.
4. Pour egg mixture into the pan and bake for 20 minutes.
5. Slice and serve.

Nutritions: *Calories 115, Fat 7g, Carbohydrates 1g, Sugar 1g, Protein 10g, Cholesterol 250 mg*

79. PORK MEATLOAF

PREPARATION: 10 MIN

COOKING: 50 MIN

SERVES: 8

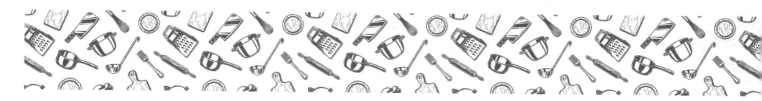

INGREDIENTS

- 95% lean ground beef – 1 pound
- Breadcrumbs – ½ cup
- Chopped sweet onion – ½ cup
- Egg – 1
- Chopped fresh basil – 2 Tbsps.
- Chopped fresh thyme -1 tsp.
- Chopped fresh parsley – 1 tsp.
- Ground black pepper – ¼ tsp.
- Brown sugar – 1 Tbsp.
- White vinegar – 1 tsp.
- Garlic powder – ¼ tsp.

DIRECTIONS

1. Preheat the oven to 350F.
2. Mix together the breadcrumbs, beef, onion, basil, egg, thyme, parsley, and pepper until well combined.
3. Press the meat mixture into a 9-by-4-inch loaf pan.
4. In a bowl, stir together the brown sugar, vinegar, and garlic powder.
5. Spread the brown sugar mixture over the meat.
6. Bake the meatloaf for about 50 minutes or until it is cooked through.
7. Let the meatloaf stand for 10 min and then pour out any accumulated grease.

Nutritions: *Calories: 103, Fat: 3g, Carb: 7g, Phosphorus: 112mg, Potassium: 190mg, Sodium: 87mg, Protein: 11g*

80. CHICKEN STEW

PREPARATION: 20 MIN

COOKING: 50 MIN

SERVES: 6

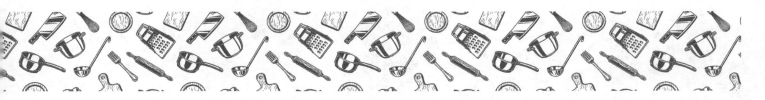

INGREDIENTS

- Olive oil – 1 Tbsp.
- Boneless, skinless chicken thighs – 1 pound, cut into 1-inch cubes
- Sweet onion – ½, chopped
- Minced garlic – 1 Tbsp.
- Chicken stock – 2 cups
- Water – 1 cup, plus 2 Tbsps.
- Carrot – 1, sliced
- Celery – 2 stalks, sliced
- Turnip – 1, sliced thin
- Chopped fresh thyme – 1 Tbsp.
- Chopped fresh rosemary – 1 tsp.
- Cornstarch – 2 tsps.
- Ground black pepper to taste

DIRECTIONS

1. Place a large saucepan on average heat and add the olive oil.
2. Sauté the chicken for 6 minutes or until it is lightly browned, stirring often.
3. Add the onion and garlic, and sauté for 3 minutes.
4. Add 1-cup water, chicken stock, carrot, celery, and turnip and bring the stew to a boil.
5. Reduce the heat to low and boil for 30 minutes or until the chicken is cooked through and tender.
6. Add the thyme and rosemary and simmer for 3 minutes more.
7. In a small bowl, stir together the 2 tbsps. Of water and the cornstarch; add the mixture to the stew.
8. Stir to incorporate the cornstarch mixture and cook for 3 to 4 minutes or until the stew thickens.
9. Remove from the heat and season with pepper.

Nutritions: *Calories: 141, Fat: 8g, Carb: 5g, Phosphorus: 53mg, Potassium: 192mg, Sodium: 214mg, Protein: 9g*

81. BEEF CHILI

PREPARATION: 10 MIN

COOKING: 30 MIN

SERVES: 2

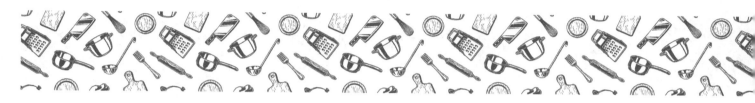

INGREDIENTS

- Onion – 1, diced
- Red bell pepper – 1, diced
- Garlic – 2 cloves, minced
- Lean ground beef – 6 oz.
- Chili powder – 1 tsp.
- Oregano – 1 tsp.
- Extra virgin olive oil – 2 Tbsps.
- Water – 1 cup
- Brown rice -1 cup
- Fresh cilantro – 1 Tbsp. to serve

DIRECTIONS

1. Soak vegetables in warm water.
2. Bring a pan of water and add rice for 20 minutes.
3. Meanwhile, add the oil to a pan and heat on medium-high heat.
4. Add the pepper, onions, and garlic and sauté for 5 minutes until soft.
5. Remove and set aside.
6. Add the beef to the pan and stir until browned.
7. Add the vegetables into the pan and stir.
8. Now add the chili powder and herbs and the water, cover and turn the heat down a little to simmer for 15 minutes.
9. Meanwhile, drain the water from the rice, and the lid and steam while the chili is cooking.
10. Serve hot with the fresh cilantro sprinkled over the top.

Nutritions: *Calories: 459, Fat: 22g, Carb: 36g, Phosphorus: 332mg, Potassium: 360mg, Sodium: 33mg, Protein: 22g*

82. SHRIMP PAELLA

PREPARATION: 5 MIN

COOKING: 10 MIN

SERVES: 2

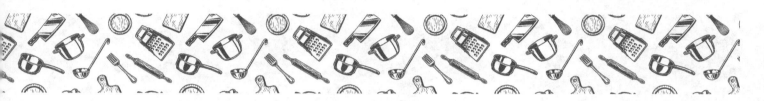

INGREDIENTS

- 1 cup cooked brown rice
- 1 chopped red onion
- 1 tsp. paprika
- 1 chopped garlic clove
- 1 tbsp. olive oil
- 6 oz. frozen cooked shrimp
- 1 deseeded and sliced chili pepper
- 1 tbsp. oregano

DIRECTIONS

1. Heat olive oil in a large pan on medium-high heat.
2. Add the onion and garlic and sauté for 2-3 minutes until soft.
3. Now add the shrimp and sauté for a further 5 minutes or until hot through.
4. Now add the herbs, spices, chili and rice with 1/2 cup boiling water.
5. Stir until everything is warm and the water has been absorbed.
6. Plate up and serve.

Nutritions: *Calories 221,Protein 17 g, Carbs 31 g, Fat 8 g, Sodium (Na) 235 mg, Potassium (K) 176 mg, Phosphorus 189 mg*

83. SALMON & PESTO SALAD

PREPARATION: 5 MIN

COOKING: 15 MIN

SERVES: 2

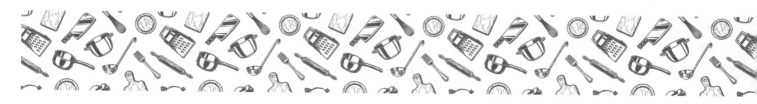

INGREDIENTS

For the pesto:
- 1 minced garlic clove
- ½ cup fresh arugula
- ¼ cup extra virgin olive oi l
- ½ cup fresh basil
- 1 tsp. black pepper
- For the salmon:
- 4 oz. skinless salmon fillet
- 1 tbsp. coconut oil

For the salad:
- ½ juiced lemon
- 2 sliced radishes
- ½ cup iceberg lettuce
- 1 tsp. black pepper

DIRECTIONS

1. Add a skillet to the stove on medium-high heat and melt the coconut oil.
2. Add the salmon to the pan.
3. Cook for 7-8 minutes and turn over.
4. Remove fillets from the skillet and allow to rest.
5. Mix the lettuce and the radishes and squeeze over the juice of ½ lemon.
6. Flake the salmon with a fork and mix through the salad.
7. Toss to coat and sprinkle with a little black pepper to serve.

Nutritions: Calories 221, Protein 13 g, Carbs 1 g, Fat 34 g, Sodium (Na) 80 mg, Potassium (K) 119 mg, Phosphorus 158 mg

84. BAKED FENNEL & GARLIC SEA BASS

PREPARATION: 5 MIN

COOKING: 15 MIN

SERVES: 2

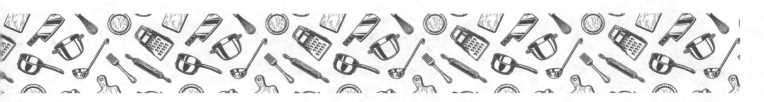

INGREDIENTS

- 1 lemon
- ½ sliced fennel bulb
- 6 oz. sea bass fillets
- 1 tsp. black pepper
- 2 garlic cloves

DIRECTIONS

1. Preheat the oven to 375°/Gas Mark 5.
2. Sprinkle black pepper over the Sea Bass.
3. Slice the fennel bulb and garlic cloves.
4. Add 1 salmon fillet and half the fennel and garlic to one sheet of baking paper or tin foil.
5. Squeeze in 1/2 lemon juices.
6. Repeat for the other fillet.
7. Fold and add to the oven for 12-15 minutes or until fish is thoroughly cooked through.
8. Meanwhile, add boiling water to your couscous, cover and allow to steam.
9. Serve with your choice of rice or salad.

Nutritions: *Calories 221, Protein 14 g, Carbs 3 g, Fat 2 g, Sodium (Na) 119 mg, Potassium (K) 398 mg, Phosphorus 149 mg*

85. LEMON, GARLIC & CILANTRO TUNA AND RICE

PREPARATION: 5 MIN

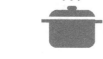
COOKING: 0 MIN

SERVES: 2

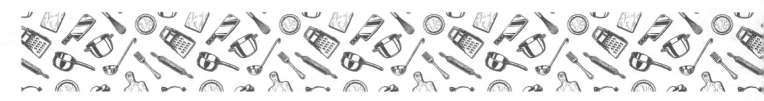

INGREDIENTS

- ½ cup arugula
- 1 tbsp. extra virgin olive oil
- 1 cup cooked rice
- 1 tsp. black pepper
- ¼ finely diced red onion
- 1 juiced lemon
- 3 oz. canned tuna
- 2 tbsps. Chopped fresh cilantro

DIRECTIONS

1. Mix the olive oil, pepper, cilantro and red onion in a bowl.
2. Stir in the tuna, cover and leave in the fridge for as long as possible (if you can) or serve immediately.
3. When ready to eat, serve up with the cooked rice and arugula!

Nutritions: *Calories 221, Protein 11 g, Carbs 26 g, Fat 7 g, Sodium (Na) 143 mg, Potassium (K)197 mg, Phosphorus 182 mg*

86. COD & GREEN BEAN RISOTTO

PREPARATION: 4 MIN

COOKING: 40 MIN

SERVES: 2

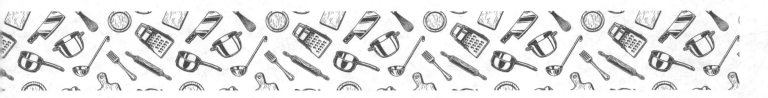

INGREDIENTS

- ½ cup arugula
- 1 finely diced white onion
- 4 oz. c od fillet
- 1 cup white rice
- 2 lemon wedges
- 1 cup boiling water
- ¼ tsp. black pepper
- 1 cup low sodium chicken broth
- 1 tbsp. extra virgin olive oil
- ½ cup green beans

DIRECTIONS

1. Heat oil in a large pan on medium heat.
2. Sauté the chopped onion for 5 minutes until soft before adding in the rice and stirring for 1-2 minutes.
3. Combine the broth with boiling water.
4. Add half of the liquid to the pan and stir slowly.
5. Slowly add the rest of the liquid whilst continuously stirring for up to 20-30 minutes.
6. Stir in the green beans to the risotto.
7. Place the fish on top of the rice, cover and steam for 10 minutes.
8. Ensure the water does not dry out and keep topping up until the rice is cooked thoroughly.
9. Use your fork to break up the fish fillets and stir into the rice.
10. Sprinkle with freshly ground pepper to serve and a squeeze of fresh lemon.
11. Garnish with the lemon wedges and serve with the arugula.

Nutritions: *Calories 221, Protein 12 g, Carbs 29 g, Fat 8 g, Sodium (Na) 398 mg, Potassium (K) 347 mg, Phosphorus 241 mg*

87. SARDINE FISH CAKES

PREPARATION: 10 MIN

COOKING: 10 MIN

SERVES: 4

INGREDIENTS

- 11 oz sardines, canned, drained
- 1/3 cup shallot, chopped
- 1 teaspoon chili flakes
- ½ teaspoon salt
- 2 tablespoon wheat flour, whole grain
- 1 egg, beaten
- 1 tablespoon chives, chopped
- 1 teaspoon olive oil
- 1 teaspoon butter

DIRECTIONS

1. Put butter in the skillet and melt it.
2. Add shallot and cook it until translucent.
3. After this, transfer the shallot in the mixing bowl.
4. Add sardines, chili flakes, salt, flour, egg, chives, and mix up until smooth with the help of the fork.
5. Make the medium size cakes and place them in the skillet.
6. Add olive oil.
7. Roast the fish cakes for 3 minutes from each side over the medium heat.
8. Dry the cooked fish cakes with the paper towel if needed and transfer in the serving plates.

Nutritions: *Calories 221, Fat 12.2, Fiber 0.1, Carbs 5.4, Protein 21.3*

88. CAJUN CATFISH

PREPARATION: 10 MIN

COOKING: 10 MIN

SERVES: 4

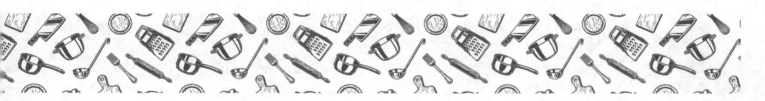

INGREDIENTS

- 16 oz catfish steaks (4 oz each fish steak)
- 1 tablespoon Cajun spices
- 1 egg, beaten
- 1 tablespoon sunflower oil

DIRECTIONS

1. Pour sunflower oil in the skillet and preheat it until shimmering.
2. Meanwhile, dip every catfish steak in the beaten egg and coat in Cajun spices.
3. Place the fish steaks in the hot oil and roast them for 4 minutes from each side.
4. The cooked catfish steaks should have a light brown crust.

Nutritions: *Calories 263, Fat 16.7, Fiber 0, Carbs 0.1, Protein 26.3*

89. 4-INGREDIENTS SALMON FILLET

PREPARATION: 5 MIN

COOKING: 25 MIN

SERVES: 1

INGREDIENTS

- 4 oz salmon fillet
- ½ teaspoon salt
- 1 teaspoon sesame oil
- ½ teaspoon sage

DIRECTIONS

1. Rub the fillet with salt and sage.
2. Place fish in the tray and sprinkle it with sesame oil.
3. Cook the fish for 25 minutes at 365F.
4. Flip the fish carefully onto another side after 12 minutes of cooking.

Nutritions: *Calories 191, Fat 11.6, Fiber 0.1, Carbs 0.2, Protein 22*

90. SPANISH COD IN SAUCE

PREPARATION: 10 MIN

COOKING: 5.5 H

SERVES: 2

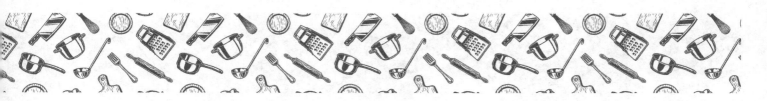

INGREDIENTS

- 1 teaspoon tomato paste
- 1 teaspoon garlic, diced
- 1 white onion, sliced
- 1 jalapeno pepper, chopped
- 1/3 cup chicken stock
- 7 oz Spanish cod fillet
- 1 teaspoon paprika
- 1 teaspoon salt

DIRECTIONS

1. Pour chicken stock in the saucepan.
2. Add tomato paste and mix up the liquid until homogenous.
3. Add garlic, onion, jalapeno pepper, paprika, and salt.
4. Bring the liquid to boil and then simmer it.
5. Chop the cod fillet and add it in the tomato liquid.
6. Close the lid and simmer the fish for 10 minutes over the low heat.
7. Serve the fish in the bowls with tomato sauce.

Nutritions: *Calories 113, Fat 1.2, Fiber 1.9, Carbs 7.2, Protein 18.9*

91. FISH SHAKSHUKA

PREPARATION: 5 MIN **COOKING: 15 MIN** **SERVES: 5**

INGREDIENTS

- 5 eggs
- 1 cup tomatoes, chopped
- 3 bell peppers, chopped
- 1 tablespoon butter
- 1 teaspoon tomato paste
- 1 teaspoon chili pepper
- 1 teaspoon salt
- 1 tablespoon fresh dill
- 5 oz cod fillet, chopped
- 1 tablespoon scallions, chopped

DIRECTIONS

1. Melt butter in the skillet and add chili pepper, bell peppers, and tomatoes.
2. Sprinkle the vegetables with scallions, dill, salt, and chili pepper. Simmer them for 5 minutes.
3. After this, add chopped cod fillet and mix up well.
4. Close the lid and simmer the ingredients for 5 minutes over the medium heat.
5. Then crack the eggs over fish and close the lid.
6. Cook shakshuka with the closed lid for 5 minutes.

Nutritions: *Calories 143, Fat 7.3, Fiber 1.6, Carbs 7.9, Protein 12.8*

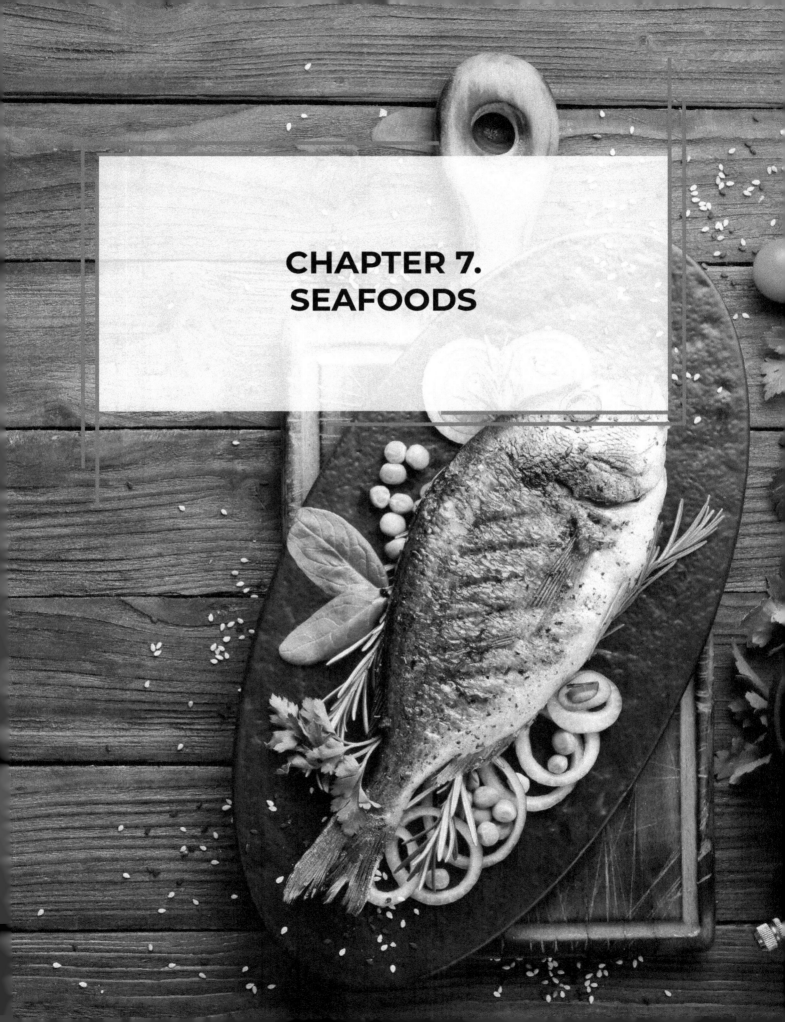

CHAPTER 7.
SEAFOODS

92. CURRIED FISH CAKES

PREPARATION: 10 MIN

COOKING: 18 MIN

SERVES: 4

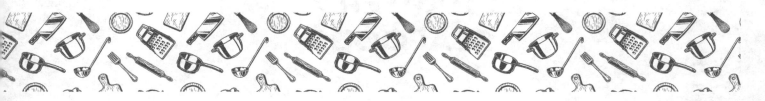

INGREDIENTS

- ¾ pound atlantic cod, cubed
- 1 apple, peeled and cubed
- 1 tablespoon yellow curry paste
- 2 tablespoons cornstarch
- 1 tablespoon peeled grated ginger root
- 1 large egg
- 1 tablespoon freshly squeezed lemon juice
- 1/8 teaspoon freshly ground black pepper
- ½ cup crushed puffed rice cereal
- 1 tablespoon olive oil

DIRECTIONS

1. Put the cod, apple, curry, cornstarch, ginger, egg, lemon juice, and pepper in a blender or food processor and process until finely chopped. Avoid over-processing, or the mixture will become mushy.
2. Place the rice cereal on a shallow plate.
3. Form the mixture into 8 patties.
4. Dredge the patties in the rice cereal to coat.
5. Cook patties for 3 to 5 minutes per side, turning once until a meat thermometer register 160°f.
6. Serve.

Nutritions: *Calories: 188; Total Fat: 6g; Saturated Fat: 1g; Sodium: 150mg; Potassium: 292mg; Phosphorus: 150mg; Carbohydrates: 12g; Fiber: 1g; Protein: 21g; Sugar: 5g*

93. BAKED SOLE WITH CARAMELIZED ONION

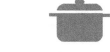

PREPARATION: 10 MIN   **COOKING: 20 MIN**   **SERVES: 4**

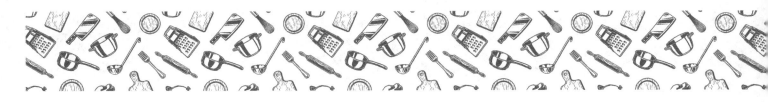

INGREDIENTS

- 1 cup finely chopped onion
- ½ cup low-sodium vegetable broth
- 1 yellow summer squash, sliced
- 2 cups frozen broccoli florets
- 4 (3-ounce) fillets of sole
- Pinch salt
- 2 tablespoons olive oil
- Pinch baking soda
- 2 teaspoons avocado oil
- 1 teaspoon dried basil leaves

DIRECTIONS

1. Preheat the oven to 425°f.
2. Add the onions. Cook for 1 minute; then, stirring constantly, cook for another 4 minutes.
3. Remove the onions from the heat.
4. Pour the broth into a baking sheet with a lip and arrange the squash and broccoli on the sheet in a single layer. Top the vegetables with the fish. Sprinkle the fish with the salt and drizzle everything with the olive oil.
5. Bake the fish and the vegetables for 10 minutes.
6. While the fish is baking, return the skillet with the onions to medium-high heat and stir in a pinch of baking soda. Stir in the avocado oil and cook for 5 minutes, stirring frequently, until the onions are dark brown.
7. Transfer the onions to a plate.
8. Tp the fish evenly with the onions. Sprinkle with the basil.
9. Return the fish to the oven, after this bake it 8 to10 minutes serve the fish on the vegetables.

Nutritions: *Calories: 202; Total Fat: 11g; Saturated Fat: 3g; Sodium: 320mg; Potassium: 537; Phosphorus: 331mg; Carbohydrates: 10g; Fiber: 3g; Protein: 16g; Sugar: 4g*

94. THAI TUNA WRAPS

PREPARATION: 10 MIN

COOKING: 0 MIN

SERVES: 4

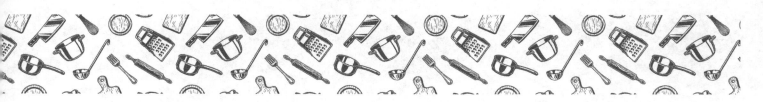

INGREDIENTS

- ¼ cup unsalted peanut butter
- 2 tablespoons freshly squeezed lemon juice
- 1 teaspoon low-sodium soy sauce
- ½ teaspoon ground ginger
- 1/8 teaspoon cayenne pepper
- 1 (6-ounce) can no-salt-added or low-sodium chunk light tuna, drained
- 1 cup shredded red cabbage
- 2 scallions, white and green parts, chopped
- 1 cup grated carrots
- 8 butter lettuce leaves

DIRECTIONS

1. In a bowl, stir together the peanut butter, lemon juice, soy sauce, ginger, and cayenne pepper until well combined.
2. Stir in the tuna, cabbage, scallions, and carrots.
3. Divide the tuna filling evenly between the butter lettuce leaves and serve.

Nutritions: *Calories: 175; Total Fat; 10g; Saturated Fat: 1g; Sodium: 98mg; Potassium: 421mg; Phosphorus: 153mg; Carbohydrates: 8g; Fiber: 2g; Protein: 17g; Sugar: 4g*

95. GRILLED FISH AND VEGETABLE PACKETS

PREPARATION: 15 MIN

COOKING: 12 MIN

SERVES: 4

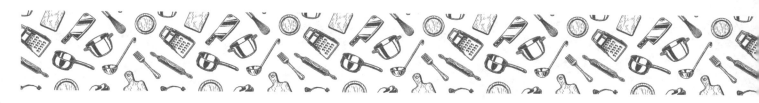

INGREDIENTS

- 1 (8-ounce) package sliced mushrooms
- 1 leek, white and green parts, chopped
- 1 cup frozen corn
- 4 (4-ounce) atlantic cod fillets
- Juice of 1 lemon
- 3 tablespoons olive oil

DIRECTIONS

1. Prepare and preheat the grill to medium coals and set a grill 6 inches from the coals.
2. Tear off four 30-inch long strips of heavy-duty aluminum foil.
3. Arrange the mushrooms, leek, and corn in the center of each piece of foil and top with the fish.
4. Drizzle the packet contents evenly with the lemon juice and olive oil.
5. Bring the longer length sides of the foil together at the top and, holding the edges together, fold them over twice and then fold in the width sides to form a sealed packet with room for the steam.
6. Put the packets on the grill and grill for 10 to 12 minutes until the vegetables are tender-crisp and the fish flakes when tested with a fork. Be careful opening the packets because the escaping steam can be scalding.

Nutritions: *Calories: 267; Total Fat: 12g; Saturated Fat: 2g; Sodium: 97mg; Potassium: 582mg; Phosphorus: 238mg; Carbohydrates: 13g; Fiber: 2g; Protein: 29g; Sugar: 3g*

96. WHITE FISH SOUP

PREPARATION: 15 MIN

COOKING: 20 MIN

SERVES: 4

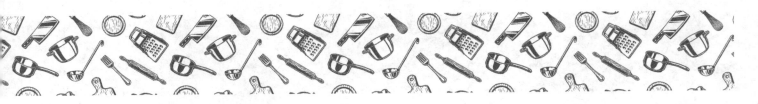

INGREDIENTS

- 2 tablespoons olive oil
- 1 onion, finely diced
- 1 green bell pepper, chopped
- 1 rib celery, thinly sliced
- 3 cups chicken broth, or more to taste
- 1/4 cup chopped fresh parsley
- 1 1/2 pounds cod, cut into 3/4-inch cubes
- Pepper to taste
- 1 dash red pepper flakes

DIRECTIONS

1. Heat oil in a soup pot over medium heat.
2. Add onion, bell pepper, and celery and cook until wilted, about 5 minutes.
3. Add broth and then bring to a simmer, about 5 minutes.
4. Cook 15 to 20 minutes.
5. Add cod, parsley, and red pepper flakes and simmer until fish flakes easily with a fork, 8 to 10 minutes more.
6. Season with black pepper.

Nutritions: *Calories 117, Total Fat 7.2g, Saturated Fat 1.4g, Cholesterol 18mg, Sodium 37mg, Total Carbohydrate 5.4g, Dietary Fiber 1.3g, Total Sugars 2.8g, Protein 8.1g, Calcium 23mg, Iron 1mg, Potassium 122mg, Phosphorus 111 Mg*

97. LEMON BUTTER SALMON

PREPARATION: 15 MIN   **COOKING: 15 MIN**   **SERVES: 6**

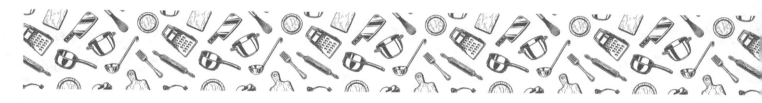

INGREDIENTS

- 1 tablespoon butter
- 2 tablespoons olive oil
- 1 tablespoon dijon mustard
- 1 tablespoons lemon juice
- 2 cloves garlic, crushed
- 1 teaspoon dried dill
- 1 teaspoon dried basil leaves
- 1 tablespoon capers
- 24-ounce salmon filet

DIRECTIONS

1. Put all the ingredients except the salmon in a saucepan over medium heat.
2. Bring to a boil and then simmer for 5 minutes.
3. Preheat your grill.
4. Create a packet using foil.
5. Place the sauce and salmon inside.
6. Seal the packet.
7. Grill for 12 minutes.

Nutritions: *Calories 292, Protein 22g, Carbohydrates 2g, Fat 22g, Cholesterol 68mg, Sodium 190mg, Potassium 439mg, Phosphorus 280mg, Calcium 21mg*

98. CRAB CAKE

PREPARATION: 15 MIN

COOKING: 9 MIN

SERVES: 6

INGREDIENTS

- 1/4 cup onion, chopped
- 1/4 cup bell pepper, chopped
- 1 egg, beaten
- 6 low-sodium crackers, crushed
- 1/4 cup low-fat mayonnaise
- 1-pound crab meat
- 1 tablespoon dry mustard
- Pepper to taste
- 2 tablespoons lemon juice
- 1 tablespoon fresh parsley
- 1 tablespoon garlic powder
- 3 tablespoons olive oil

DIRECTIONS

1. Mix all the ingredients except the oil.
2. Form 6 patties from the mixture.
3. Pour the oil into a pan in a medium heat.
4. Cook the crab cakes for 5 minutes.
5. Flip and cook for another 4 minutes.

Nutritions: *Calories 189, Protein 13g, Carbohydrates 5g, Fat 14g, Cholesterol 111mg, Sodium 342mg, Potassium 317mg, Phosphorus 185mg, Calcium 52mg, Fiber 0.5g*

99. BAKED FISH IN CREAM SAUCE

PREPARATION: 10 MIN

COOKING: 40 MIN

SERVES: 4

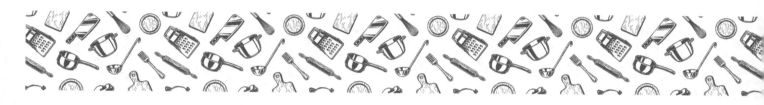

INGREDIENTS

- 1-pound haddock
- 1/2 cup all-purpose flour
- 2 tablespoons butter (unsalted)
- 1/4 teaspoon pepper
- 2 cups fat-free nondairy creamer
- 1/4 cup water

DIRECTIONS

1. Preheat your oven to 350 degrees f.
2. Spray baking pan with oil.
3. Sprinkle with a little flour.
4. Arrange fish on the pan
5. Season with pepper.
6. Sprinkle remaining flour on the fish.
7. Spread creamer on both sides of the fish.
8. Bake for 40 minutes or until golden.
9. Spread cream sauce on top of the fish before serving.

Nutritions: *Calories 383, Protein 24g, Carbohydrates 46g, Fat 11g, Cholesterol 79mg, Sodium 253mg, Potassium 400mg, Phosphorus 266mg, Calcium 46mg, Fiber 0.4g*

100. SHRIMP & BROCCOLI

PREPARATION: 10 MIN

COOKING: 5 MIN

SERVES: 4

INGREDIENTS

- 1 tablespoon olive oil
- 1 clove garlic, minced
- 1-pound shrimp
- 1/4 cup red bell pepper
- 1 cup broccoli florets, steamed
- 10-ounce cream cheese
- 1/2 teaspoon garlic powder
- 1/4 cup lemon juice
- 3/4 teaspoon ground peppercorns
- 1/4 cup half and half creamer

DIRECTIONS

1. Pour the oil and cook garlic for 30 seconds.
2. Add shrimp and cook for 2 minutes.
3. Add the rest of the ingredients.
4. Mix well.
5. Cook for 2 minutes.

Nutritions: *Calories 469, Protein 28g, Carbohydrates 28g, Fat 28g, Cholesterol 213mg, Sodium 374mg, Potassium 469mg, Phosphorus 335mg, Calcium 157mg, Fiber 2.6g*

101. SHRIMP IN GARLIC SAUCE

PREPARATION: 10 MIN   **COOKING: 6 MIN**   **SERVES: 4**

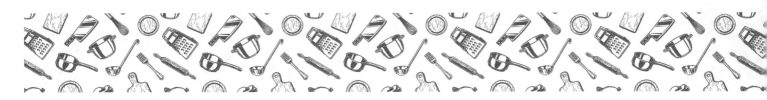

INGREDIENTS

- 3 tablespoons butter (unsalted)
- 1/4 cup onion, minced
- 3 cloves garlic, minced
- 1-pound shrimp, shelled and deveined
- 1/2 cup half and half creamer
- 1/4 cup white wine
- 2 tablespoons fresh basil
- Black pepper to taste

DIRECTIONS

1. Add butter to a pan over medium low heat.
2. Let it melt.
3. Add the onion and garlic.
4. Cook for it 1-2 minutes.
5. Add shrimp and cook for 2 minutes.
6. Transfer shrimp on a serving platter and set aside.
7. Add the rest of the ingredients.
8. Simmer for 3 minutes.
9. Pour sauce over the shrimp and serve.

Nutritions: Calories 482, Protein 33g, Carbohydrates 46g, Fat 11g, Cholesterol 230mg, Sodium 213mg, Potassium 514mg, Phosphorus 398mg, Calcium 133mg, Fiber 2.0g

102. FISH TACO

PREPARATION: 40 MIN

COOKING: 10 MIN

SERVES: 6

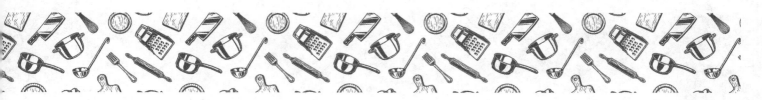

INGREDIENTS

- 1 tablespoon lime juice
- 1 tablespoon olive oil
- 1 clove garlic, minced
- 1-pound cod fillets
- 1/2 teaspoon ground cumin
- 1/4 teaspoon black pepper
- 1/2 teaspoon chili powder
- 1/4 cup sour cream
- 1/2 cup mayonnaise
- 2 tablespoons nondairy milk
- 1 cup cabbage, shredded
- 1/2 cup onion, chopped
- 1/2 bunch cilantro, chopped
- 12 corn tortillas

DIRECTIONS

1. Drizzle lemon juice over the fish fillet.
2. Coat it with olive oil and then season with garlic, cumin, pepper and chili powder.
3. Let it sit for 30 minutes.
4. Broil fish for 10 minutes, flipping halfway through.
5. Flake the fish using a fork.
6. In a bowl, mix sour cream, milk and mayo.
7. Assemble tacos by filling each tortilla with mayo mixture, cabbage, onion, cilantro and fish flakes.

Nutritions: *Calories 366, Protein 18g, Carbohydrates 31g, Fat 19g, Cholesterol 40mg, Sodium 194mg, Potassium 507mg, Phosphorus 327mg, Calcium 138mg, Fiber 4.3g*

103. BAKED TROUT

PREPARATION: 5 MIN

COOKING: 10 MIN

SERVES: 8

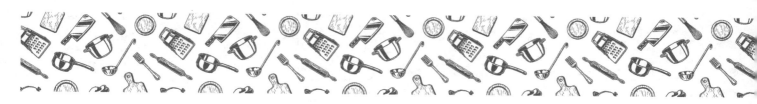

INGREDIENTS

- 2-pound trout fillet
- 1 tablespoon oil
- 1 teaspoon salt-free lemon pepper
- 1/2 teaspoon paprika

DIRECTIONS

1. Preheat your oven to 350 degrees f.
2. Coat fillet with oil.
3. Place fish on a baking pan.
4. Season with lemon pepper and paprika.
5. Bake for 10 minutes.

Nutritions: *Calories 161, Protein 21g, Carbohydrates 0g, Fat 8g, Cholesterol 58mg, Sodium 109mg, Potassium 385mg, Phosphorus 227mg, Calcium 75mg, Fiber 0.1g*

104. FISH WITH MUSHROOMS

PREPARATION: 5 MIN

COOKING: 16 MIN

SERVES: 4

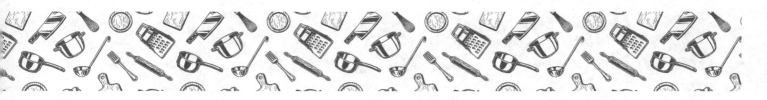

INGREDIENTS

- 1-pound cod fillet
- 2 tablespoons butter
- ¼ cup white onion, chopped
- 1 cup fresh mushrooms
- 1 teaspoon dried thyme

DIRECTIONS

1. Put the fish in a baking pan.
2. Preheat your oven to 450 degrees f.
3. Melt the butter and cook onion and mushroom for 1 minute.
4. Spread mushroom mixture on top of the fish.
5. Season with thyme.
6. Bake in the oven for 15 minutes.

Nutritions: *Calories 156, Protein 21g, Carbohydrates 3g, Fat 7g, Cholesterol 49mg, Sodium 110mg, Potassium 561mg, Phosphorus 225mg, Calcium 30mg, Fiber 0.5g*

105. SALMON WITH SPICY HONEY

PREPARATION: 15 MIN

COOKING: 8 MIN

SERVES: 2

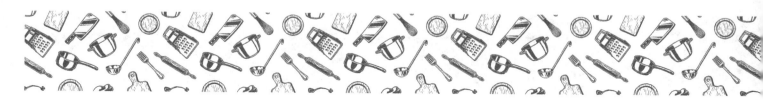

INGREDIENTS

- 16-ounce salmon fillet
- 3 tablespoon honey
- 3/4 teaspoon lemon peel
- 3 bowls arugula salad
- 1/2 teaspoon black pepper
- 1/2 teaspoon garlic powder
- 2 teaspoon olive oil
- 1 teaspoon hot water

DIRECTIONS

1. Prepare a small bowl with some hot water and put in honey, grated lemon peel, ground pepper, and garlic powder.
2. Spread the mixture over salmon fillets.
3. Warm some olive oil at a medium heat and add spiced salmon fillet and cook for 4 minutes.
4. Turn the fillets on one side then on the other side.
5. Continue to cook for other 4 minutes at a reduced heat and try to check when the salmon fillets flake easily.
6. Put some arugula on each plate and add the salmon fillets on top, adding some aromatic herbs or some dill. Serve and enjoy!

Nutritions: *Calories: 320 Protein: 23g Sodium: 65mg Potassium: 450mg Phosphorus: 250mg*

106. SALMON WITH MAPLE GLAZE

PREPARATION: 15 MIN

COOKING: 2 H

SERVES: 4

INGREDIENTS

- 1-pound salmon fillets
- 1 tablespoon green onion, chopped
- 1 tablespoon low sodium soy sauce
- 2 garlic cloves, pressed
- 2 tablespoon fresh cilantro
- 3 tablespoon lemon juice(or juice of 1 lemon)
- 3 tablespoon maple syrup

DIRECTIONS

1. Combine all ingredients except for salmon.
2. Put salmon on platter and then pour marinade over fillets. Let it marinate 2 hours or more.
3. Preheat broiler.
4. Remove salmon from marinade.
5. Place salmon on bottom rack and broil for 10 minutes. Do not turn over.
6. Serve hot/cold with a wedge of lemon.

Nutritions: *Calories: 220; Carbs: 12g; Protein: 24g; Fats: 8g; Phosphorus: 374mg; Potassium: 440mg; Sodium: 621mg*

107. STEAMED SPICY TILAPIA FILLET

PREPARATION: 10 MIN

COOKING: 25 MIN

SERVES: 4

INGREDIENTS

- 4 fillets of tilapia
- 1 teaspoon hot pepper sauce
- 1 large sprig thyme
- 1 tablespoon ketchup
- 1 tablespoon lime juice
- 1 cup hot water
- 1/2 cup onion, sliced
- 1/4 teaspoon black pepper
- 3/4 cup red and green peppers, sliced

DIRECTIONS

1. In a large shallow dish that fits your steamer, mix well hot pepper sauce, thyme, ketchup, lemon juice, and black pepper. Mix thoroughly.
2. Add tilapia fillets and spoon over sauce.
3. Mix in remaining ingredients except for water. Mix well in sauce.
4. Cover top of dish with foil.
5. Add the hot water in the steamer. Place dish on steamer rack. Cover pot and steam fish and veggies for 20 minutes.
6. Let it stand for 5-6 minutes before serving.

Nutritions: *Calories: 131; Carbs: 5g; Protein: 24g; Fats: 3g; Phosphorus: 212mg; Potassium: 457mg; Sodium: 102mg*

108. DIJON MUSTARD AND LIME MARINATED SHRIMP

PREPARATION: 20 MIN

COOKING: 80 MIN

SERVES: 8

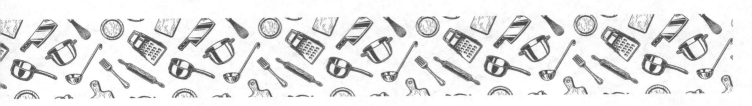

INGREDIENTS

- 1-pound uncooked shrimp, peeled and deveined
- 1 bay leaf
- 3 whole cloves
- ½ cup rice vinegar
- 1 cup water
- ½ teaspoon hot sauce
- 2 tablespoons. Capers
- 2 tablespoons. Dijon mustard
- ½ cup fresh lime juice, plus lime as garnish
- 1 medium red onion, chopped

DIRECTIONS

1. Mix hot sauce, mustard, capers, lime juice and onion in a shallow baking dish and set aside.
2. Bring it to a boil in a large saucepan bay leaf, cloves, vinegar and water.
3. Once boiling, add shrimps and cook for a minute while stirring continuously.
4. Drain shrimps and pour shrimps into onion mixture.
5. For an hour, refrigerate while covered the shrimps.
6. Then serve shrimps cold and garnished with lime zest.

Nutritions: *Calories: 123; Carbs: 3g; Protein: 12g; Fats: 1g; Phosphorus: 119mg; Potassium: 87mg; Sodium: 568mg*

109. BAKED COD CRUSTED WITH HERBS

PREPARATION: 15 MIN   COOKING: 10 MIN   SERVES: 4

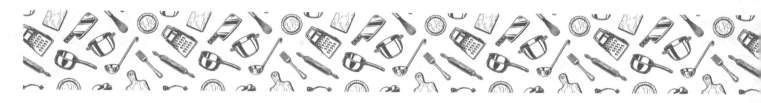

INGREDIENTS

- ¼ cup honey
- ½ cup panko
- ½ teaspoon pepper
- 1 tablespoon extra-virgin olive oil
- 1 tablespoon lemon juice
- 1 teaspoon dried basil
- 1 teaspoon dried parsley
- 1 teaspoon rosemary
- 4 pieces of 4-ounce cod fillets

DIRECTIONS

1. With olive oil, grease a 9 x 13-inch baking pan and preheat oven to 375of.
2. In a zip top bag mix panko, rosemary, pepper, parsley and basil.
3. Evenly spread cod fillets in prepped dish and drizzle with lemon juice.
4. Then brush the fillets with honey on all sides. Discard remaining honey if any.
5. Then evenly divide the panko mixture on top of cod fillets.
6. Pop in the oven and bake for ten minutes or until fish is cooked.
7. Serve and enjoy.

Nutritions: *Calories: 113; Carbs: 21g; Protein: 5g; Fats: 2g; Phosphorus: 89mg; Potassium: 115mg; Sodium: 139mg*

110. DILL RELISH ON WHITE SEA BASS

PREPARATION: 15 MIN

COOKING: 60 MIN

SERVES: 4

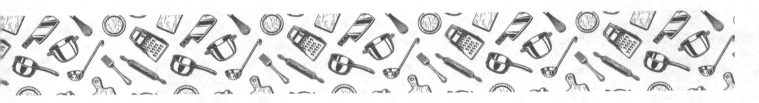

INGREDIENTS

- 1 lemon, quartered
- 4 pieces of 4-ounce white sea bass fillets
- 1 teaspoon lemon juice
- 1 teaspoon dijon mustard
- 1 ½ teaspoons. Chopped fresh dill
- 1 teaspoon pickled baby capers, drained
- 1 ½ tablespoons. Chopped white onion

DIRECTIONS

1. Preheat oven to 375of.
2. Mix lemon juice, mustard, dill, capers and onions in a small bowl.
3. Prepare four aluminum foil squares and place 1 fillet per foil.
4. Squeeze a lemon wedge per fish.
5. Evenly divide into 4 the dill spread and drizzle over fillet.
6. Close the foil over the fish securely and pop in the oven.
7. Bake for 9 to 12 minutes or until fish is cooked through.
8. Remove from foil and transfer to a serving platter, serve and enjoy.

Nutritions: *Calories: 71; Carbs: 11g; Protein: 7g; Fats: 1g; Phosphorus: 91mg; Potassium: 237mg; Sodium: 94mg*

111. TILAPIA WITH LEMON GARLIC SAUCE

PREPARATION: 15 MIN

COOKING: 30 MIN

SERVES: 4

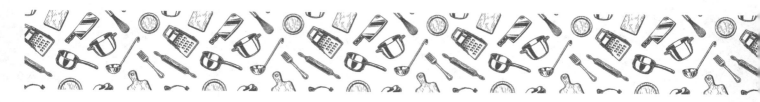

INGREDIENTS

- Pepper
- 1 teaspoon dried parsley flakes
- 1 clove garlic (finely chopped)
- 1 tablespoon butter (melted)
- 3 tablespoons. Fresh lemon juice
- 4 tilapia fillets

DIRECTIONS

1. First, spray baking dish with non-stick cooking spray then preheat oven at 375 degrees Fahrenheit (190oc).
2. In cool water, rinse tilapia fillets and using paper towels pat dry the fillets.
3. Place tilapia fillets in the baking dish then pour butter and lemon juice and top off with pepper, parsley and garlic.
4. Bake tilapia in the preheated oven for 30 minutes and wait until fish is white.
5. Enjoy!

Nutritions: *Calories: 168; Carbs: 4g; Protein: 24g; Fats: 5g; Phosphorus: 207mg; Potassium: 431mg; Sodium: 85mg*

112. SPINACH WITH TUSCAN WHITE BEANS AND SHRIMPS

PREPARATION: 5 MIN

COOKING: 15 MIN

SERVES: 4

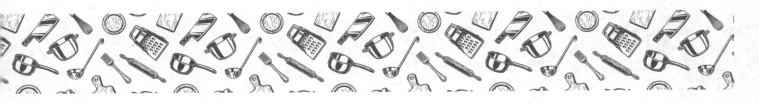

INGREDIENTS

- 1 ½ ounces crumbled reduce-fat feta cheese
- 5 cups baby spinach
- 15 ounces can no salt added cannellini beans (rinsed and drained)
- ½ cup low sodium, fat-free chicken broth
- 2 tablespoons. Balsamic vinegar
- 2 teaspoons. Chopped fresh sage
- 4 cloves garlic (minced)
- 1 medium onion (chopped)
- 1-pound large shrimp (peeled and deveined)
- 2 tablespoons. Olive oil

DIRECTIONS

1. Heat 1 teaspoon oil. Heat it over medium-high.
2. Then for about 2 to 3 minutes, cook the shrimps using the heated skillet then place them on a plate. Heat on the same skillet the sage, garlic, and onions then cook for about 4 minutes. Add and stir in vinegar for 30 seconds.
3. For about 2 minutes, add chicken broth. Then, add spinach and beans and cook for an additional 2 to 3 minutes.
4. Remove skillet then add and stir in cooked shrimps topped with feta cheese.
5. Serve and divide into 4 bowls. Enjoy!

Nutritions: *Calories: 343; Carbs: 21g; Protein: 22g; Fats: 11g; Phosphorus: 400mg; Potassium: 599mg; Sodium: 766mg*

113. BAGEL WITH SALMON AND EGG

PREPARATION: 15 MIN

COOKING: 10 MIN

SERVES: 1

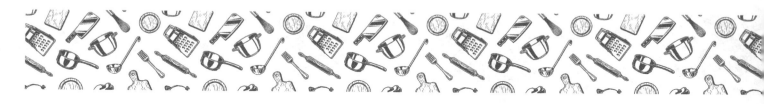

INGREDIENTS

- Bagel – ½
- Cream cheese – 1 tablespoon
- Scallions – 1 tablespoon
- Fresh dill – ½ teaspoon
- Fresh basil leaves – 2
- Tomato – 1 slice
- Arugula – 4 pieces
- Egg – 1 large
- Cooked salmon – 1 ounce

DIRECTIONS

1. Start by slicing the bagel through the center horizontally. Take one half of the bagel and toast it in an oven or a toaster.
2. Finely chop the dill, basil leaves, and scallions. Set aside.
3. Add in the cream cheese. Toss in the chopped dill, basil, and scallions. Mix well to combine. Take the toasted bagel and spread the herbs and cream cheese mixture evenly over it.
4. Place the tomato slice and arugula on top. Set aside.
5. Take a small mixing bowl and then beat the egg.
6. Take a non-stick saucepan and grease it using cooking spray. Stir after pouring the beaten egg into the pan and. Cook for about 1 minute over medium heat. Keep stirring to make a perfect scrambled egg.
7. Take the cooked salmon and place it in the same pan as the egg. This will help you heat the salmon and cook the egg at the same time.
8. Place the scrambled egg over the tomato slice and top it with the salmon.

Nutritions: *Protein 19g, Fat 14g, Carbohydrates 29g, Cholesterol 218mg, Potassium 338mg, Sodium 378mg, Phosphorus 270mg, Fiber 2.6g, Calcium 77*

114. SALMON STUFFED PASTA

PREPARATION: 20 MIN

COOKING: 35 MIN

SERVES: 24

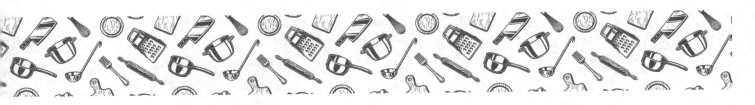

INGREDIENTS

- 24 jumbo pasta shells, boiled
- 1 cup coffee creamer

Filling:
- 2 eggs, beaten
- 2 cups creamed cottage cheese
- ¼ cup chopped onion
- 1 red bell pepper, diced
- 2 teaspoons dried parsley
- ½ teaspoon lemon peel
- 1 can salmon, drained

Dill sauce:
- 1 ½ teaspoon butter
- 1 ½ teaspoon flour
- 1/8 teaspoon pepper
- 1 tablespoon lemon juice
- 1 ½ cup coffee creamer
- 2 teaspoons dried dill weed

DIRECTIONS

1. Beat the cream cheese with the egg and all the other filling ingredients in a bowl.
2. Divide the filling in the pasta shells and place the shells in a 9x13 baking dish.
3. Pour the coffee creamer around the stuffed shells then cover with a foil.
4. Bake the shells for 30 minutes at 350 degrees f.
5. Meanwhile, whisk all the ingredients for dill sauce in a saucepan.
6. Stir for 5 minutes until it thickens.
7. Pour this sauce over the baked pasta shells.
8. Serve warm.

Nutritions: *Calories 268, Total fat 4.8g, Sodium 86mg, Protein 11.5g, Calcium 27mg, Phosphorous 314mg, Potassium 181mg*

115. HERBED VEGETABLE TROUT

PREPARATION: 15 MIN

COOKING: 15 MIN

SERVES: 4

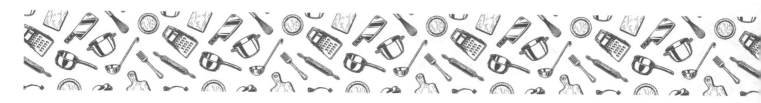

INGREDIENTS

- 14 oz. Trout fillets
- 1/2 teaspoon herb seasoning blend
- 1 lemon, sliced
- 2 green onions, sliced
- 1 stalk celery, chopped
- 1 medium carrot, julienne

DIRECTIONS

1. Prepare and preheat a charcoal grill over moderate heat.
2. Place the trout fillets over a large piece of foil and drizzle herb seasoning on top.
3. Spread the lemon slices, carrots, celery, and green onions over the fish.
4. Cover the fish with foil and pack it.
5. Place the packed fish in the grill and cook for 15 minutes.
6. Once done, remove the foil from the fish.
7. Serve.

Nutritions: *Calories 202, Total fat 8.5g, Sodium 82mg, Calcium 70mg, Phosphorous 287mg, Potassium 560mg*

116. CITRUS GLAZED SALMON

PREPARATION: 20 MIN

COOKING: 17 MIN

SERVES: 4

INGREDIENTS

- 2 garlic cloves, crushed
- 1 1/2 tablespoons lemon juice
- 2 tablespoons olive oil
- 1 tablespoon butter
- 1 tablespoon dijon mustard
- 2 dashes cayenne pepper
- 1 teaspoon dried basil leaves
- 1 teaspoon dried dill
- 24 oz. Salmon filet

DIRECTIONS

1. Place a 1-quart saucepan over moderate heat and add the oil, butter, garlic, lemon juice, mustard, cayenne pepper, dill, and basil to the pan.
2. Stir this mixture for 5 minutes after it has boiled.
3. Prepare and preheat a charcoal grill over moderate heat.
4. Place the fish on a foil sheet and fold the edges to make a foil tray.
5. Pour the prepared sauce over the fish.
6. Place the fish in the foil in the preheated grill and cook for 12 minutes.
7. Slice and serve.

Nutritions: *Calories 401, Total fat 20.5g, Cholesterol 144mg, Sodium 256mg, Carbohydrate 0.5g, Calcium 549mg, Phosphorous 214mg, Potassium 446mg*

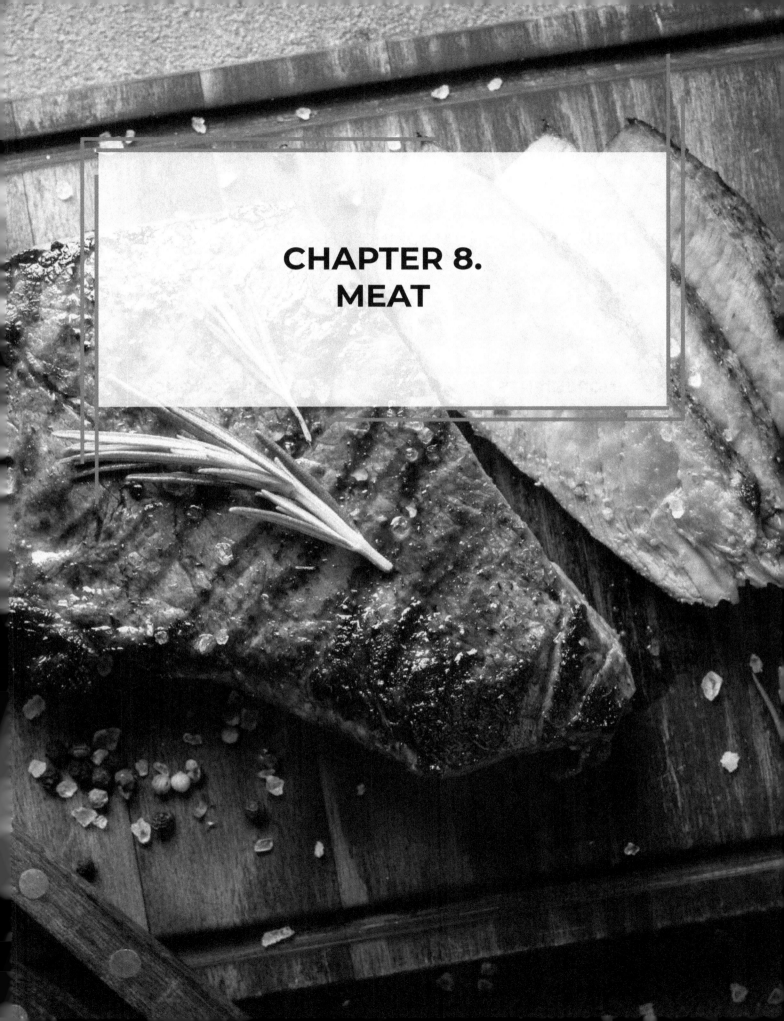

CHAPTER 8.
MEAT

117. BEEF AND THREE PEPPER STEW

PREPARATION: 15 MIN   **COOKING: 6 H**   **SERVES: 6**

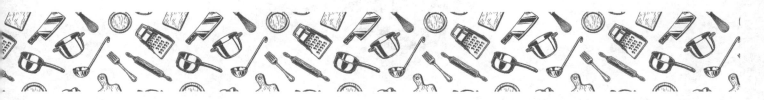

INGREDIENTS

- 10ounce of flat cut beef brisket, whole
- 1 teaspoon of dried thyme
- 1 teaspoon of black pepper
- 1 clove garlic
- ½ cup of green onion, thinly sliced
- ½ cup low sodium chicken stock
- 2 cups water
- 1 large green bell pepper, sliced
- 1 large red bell pepper, sliced
- 1 large yellow bell pepper, sliced
- 1 large red onion, sliced

DIRECTIONS

1. Combine the beef, thyme, pepper, garlic, green onion, stock and water in a slow cooker.
2. Leave it all to cook on high for 4-5 hours until tender.
3. Remove the beef from the slow cooker and let it cool.
4. Shred the beef with two forks and remove any excess fat.
5. Place the shredded beef back into the slow cooker.
6. Add the sliced peppers and the onion.
7. Cook this on high heat for 40-60 minutes until the vegetables are tender.

Nutritions: *Calories: 132, Protein: 14g, Carbohydrates: 9g, Fat: 5g, Cholesterol: 39mg, Sodium: 179mg, Potassium: 390mg, Phosphorus: 141mg, Calcium: 33mg, Fiber: 2g*

118. SPICED LAMB BURGERS

PREPARATION: 10 MIN

COOKING: 20 MIN

SERVES: 2

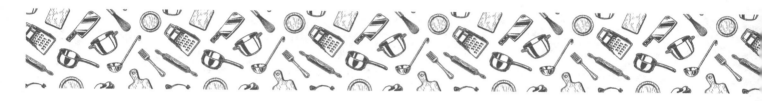

INGREDIENTS

- 1 tablespoon extra-virgin olive oil
- 1 teaspoon cumin
- ½ finely diced red onion
- 1 minced garlic clove
- 1 teaspoon harissa spices
- 1 cup arugula
- 1 juiced lemon
- 6-ounce lean ground lamb
- 1 tablespoon parsley
- ½ cup low-fat plain yogurt

DIRECTIONS

1. Preheat the broiler on a medium to high heat.
2. Mix together the ground lamb, red onion, parsley, harissa spices and olive oil until combined.
3. Shape 1-inch thick patties using wet hands.
4. Add the patties to a baking tray and place under the broiler for 7-8 minutes on each side or until thoroughly cooked through.
5. Mix the yogurt, lemon juice and cumin and serve over the lamb burgers with a side salad of arugula.

Nutritions: *Calories 306, Fat 20g, Carbs 10g, Phosphorus 269mg, Potassium (K) 492mg, Sodium (Na) 86mg, Protein 23g*

119. PORK LOINS WITH LEEKS

PREPARATION: 10 MIN

COOKING: 35 MIN

SERVES: 2

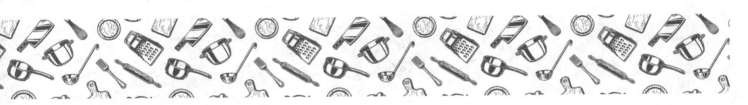

INGREDIENTS

- 1 sliced leek
- 1 tablespoon mustard seeds
- 6-ounce pork tenderloin
- 1 tablespoon cumin seeds
- 1 tablespoon dry mustard
- 1 tablespoon extra-virgin oil

DIRECTIONS

1. Preheat the broiler to medium high heat.
2. In a dry skillet heat mustard and cumin seeds until they start to pop (3-5 minutes).
3. Grind the seeds using a pestle and mortar or blender and then mix in the dry mustard.
4. Coat the pork on both sides with the mustard blend and add to a baking tray to broil for 25-30 minutes or until cooked through. Turn once halfway through.
5. Remove and place to one side.
6. Heat oil in a pan on medium heat and add the leeks for 5-6 minutes or until soft.
7. Serve the pork tenderloin on a bed of leeks and enjoy!

Nutritions: *Calories 139, Fat 5g, Carbs 2g, Phosphorus 278mg, Potassium (K) 45mg, Sodium (Na) 47mg, Protein 18g*

120. CHINESE BEEF WRAPS

PREPARATION: 10 MIN

COOKING: 30 MIN

SERVES: 2

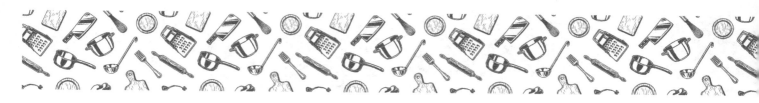

INGREDIENTS

- 2 iceberg lettuce leaves
- ½ diced cucumber
- 1 teaspoon canola oil
- 5-ounce lean ground beef
- 1 teaspoon ground ginger
- 1 tablespoon chili flakes
- 1 minced garlic clove
- 1 tablespoon rice wine vinegar

DIRECTIONS

1. Mix the ground meat with the garlic, rice wine vinegar, chili flakes and ginger in a bowl.
2. Heat oil in a skillet over medium heat.
3. Add the beef to the pan and cook for 20-25 minutes or until cooked through.
4. Serve beef mixture with diced cucumber in each lettuce wrap and fold.

Nutritions: Calories 156, Fat 2g, Carbs 4g, Phosphorus 1mg, Sodium (Na) 54mg, Protein 14g

121. GRILLED SKIRT STEAK

PREPARATION: 15 MIN

COOKING: 8-9 MIN

SERVES: 4

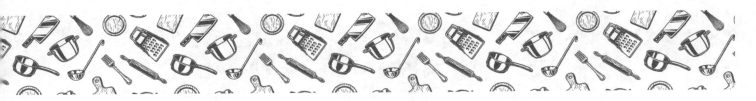

INGREDIENTS

- 2 teaspoons fresh ginger herb, grated finely
- 2 teaspoons fresh lime zest, grated finely
- ¼ cup coconut sugar
- 2 teaspoons fish sauce
- 2 tablespoons fresh lime juice
- ½ cup coconut milk
- 1-pound beef skirt steak, trimmed and cut into 4-inch slices lengthwise
- Salt, to taste

DIRECTIONS

1. In a sizable sealable bag, mix together all ingredients except steak and salt.
2. Add steak and coat with marinade generously.
3. Seal the bag and refrigerate to marinate for about 4-12 hours.
4. Preheat the grill to high heat. Grease the grill grate.
5. Remove steak from refrigerator and discard the marinade.
6. With a paper towel, dry the steak and sprinkle with salt evenly.
7. Cook the steak for approximately 3½ minutes.
8. Flip the medial side and cook for around 2½-5 minutes or till desired doneness.
9. Remove from grill pan and keep side for approximately 5 minutes before slicing.
10. With a clear, crisp knife cut into desired slices and serve.

Nutritions: *Calories: 465, Fat: 10g, Carbohydrates: 22g, Fiber: 0g, Protein: 37g*

122. LAMB WITH PRUNES

PREPARATION: 15 MIN

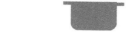

COOKING: 2 H 40 MIN

SERVES: 4-6

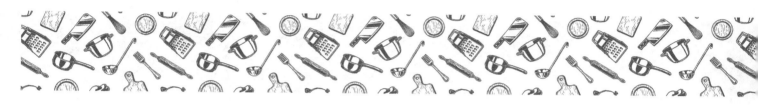

INGREDIENTS

- 3 tablespoons coconut oil
- 2 onions, chopped finely
- 1 (1-inch) piece fresh ginger, minced
- 3 garlic cloves, minced
- ½ teaspoon ground turmeric
- 2 ½ pound lamb shoulder, trimmed and cubed into 3-inch size
- Salt and freshly ground black pepper
- ½ teaspoon saffron threads, crumbled
- 1 cinnamon stick
- 3 cups water
- 1 cup runes, pitted and halved

DIRECTIONS

1. In a big pan, melt coconut oil on medium heat.
2. Add onions, ginger, garlic cloves and turmeric and sauté for about 3-5 minutes.
3. Sprinkle lamb with salt and black pepper evenly.
4. In the pan, add lamb and saffron threads and cook for approximately 4-5 minutes.
5. Add cinnamon stick and water and produce to some boil on high heat.
6. Reduce the temperature to low and simmer, covered for around 1½-120 minutes or till desired doneness of lamb.
7. Stir in prunes and simmer for approximately 20-a half-hour.
8. Remove cinnamon stick and serve hot.

Nutritions: *Calories: 393, Fat: 12g, Carbohydrates: 10g, Fiber: 4g, Protein: 36g*

123. ROAST BEEF

PREPARATION: 25 MIN

COOKING: 55 MIN

SERVES: 3

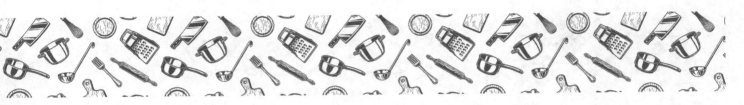

INGREDIENTS

- Quality rump or sirloin tip roast

DIRECTIONS

1. Place in roasting pan o n a shallow rack
2. Season with pepper and herbs
3. Insert meat thermometer in the center or thickest part of the roast
4. Roast to the desired degree of doneness
5. After removing from over for about 15 minutes let it chill
6. In the end the roast should be moister than well done.

Nutritions: *Calories 158 ,Protein 24g, Fat 6g, Carbs 0g, Phosphorus 206mg, Potassium (K) 328mg, Sodium (Na) 55mg*

124. BEEF BROCHETTES

PREPARATION: 20 MIN

COOKING: 1 H MIN

SERVES: 1

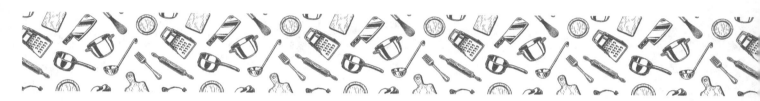

INGREDIENTS

- 1 ½ cups pineapple chunks
- 1 sliced large onion
- 2 pounds thick steak
- 1 sliced medium bell pepper
- 1 bay leaf
- ¼ cup vegetable oil
- ½ cup lemon juice
- 2 crushed garlic cloves

DIRECTIONS

1. Cut beef cubes and place in a plastic bag
2. Combine marinade ingredients in small bowl
3. Mix and pour over beef cubes
4. Seal the bag and refrigerate for 3 to 5 hours
5. Divide ingredients onion, beef cube, green pepper, pineapple
6. Grill about 9 minutes each side

Nutritions: *Calories 304, Protein 35g, Fat 15g, Carbs 11g, Phosphorus 264mg, Potassium (K) 388mg, Sodium (Na) 70mg*

125. COUNTRY FRIED STEAK

PREPARATION: 10 MIN

COOKING: 1 H 40 MIN

SERVES: 3

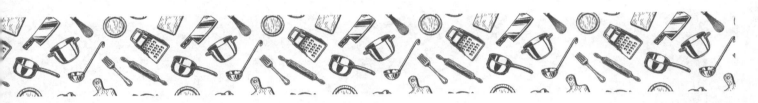

INGREDIENTS

- 1 large onion
- ½ cup flour
- 3 tablespoons. Vegetable oil
- ¼ teaspoon pepper
- 1½ pounds round steak
- ½ teaspoon paprika

DIRECTIONS

1. Trim excess fat from steak
2. Cut into small pieces
3. Combine flour, paprika and pepper and mix together
4. Preheat skillet with oil
5. Cook steak on both sides
6. When the color of steak is brown remove to a platter
7. Add water (150 ml) and stir around the skillet
8. Return browned steak to skillet, if necessary, add water again so that bottom side of steak does not stick

Nutritions: *Calories 248, Protein 30g, Fat 10g, Carbs 5g, Phosphorus 190mg, Potassium (K) 338mg, Sodium (Na) 60mg*

126. BEEF POT ROAST

PREPARATION: 20 MIN

COOKING: 1 H

SERVES: 3

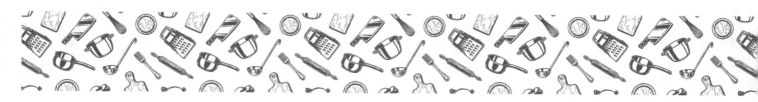

INGREDIENTS

- Round bone roast
- 2 - 4 pounds chuck roast
- Direction:
- Trim off excess fat
- Place a tablespoon of oil in a big skillet and heat to medium
- Roll pot roast in flour and brown on all sides in a hot skillet
- After the meat gets a brown color, reduce heat to low
- Season with pepper and herbs and add ½ cup of water
- Cook slowly for 1½ hours or until it looks ready

DIRECTIONS

1. Add in the pork tenderloin into a slow cooker then pour barbecue sauce over the top.
2. Cover using the lid and cook for 6 hours on medium setting until soft.
3. Remove pork tenderloin and finely shred using two forks.
4. Add in the yogurt, coleslaw, and Dijon mustard into a small-sized bowl and season using a dash of salt and black pepper. Stir until thoroughly mixed.
5. Divide pork among hamburger buns then tops off using the coleslaw.
6. Serve immediately.

Nutritions: *Calories 157, Protein 24g, Fat 13g, Carbs 0g, Phosphorus 204mg, Sodium (Na) 50mg*

127. HOMEMADE BURGERS

PREPARATION: 10 MIN

COOKING: 20 MIN

SERVES: 2

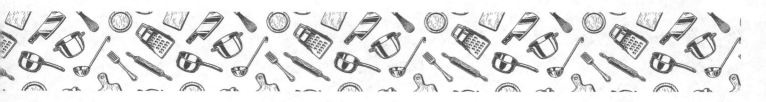

INGREDIENTS

- 4 ounce lean 100% ground beef
- 1 teaspoon black pepper
- 1 garlic clove, minced
- 1 teaspoon olive oil
- 1/4 cup onion, finely diced
- 1 tablespoon balsamic vinegar
- 1/2ounce brie cheese, crumbled
- 1 teaspoon mustard

DIRECTIONS

1. Season ground beef with pepper and then mix in minced garlic.
2. Form burger shapes with the ground beef using the palms of your hands.
3. Heat a skillet on a medium to high heat, and then add the oil.
4. Sauté the onions for 5-10 minutes until browned.
5. Then add the balsamic vinegar and sauté for another 5 minutes.
6. Remove and set aside.
7. Add the burgers to the pan and heat on the same heat for 5-6 minutes before flipping and heating for a further 5-6 minutes until cooked through.
8. Spread the mustard onto each burger.
9. Crumble the brie cheese over each burger and serve!
10. Try with a crunchy side salad!
11. Tip: if using fresh beef and not defrosted, prepare double the ingredients and freeze burgers in plastic wrap (after cooling) for up to 1 month.
12. Thoroughly defrost before heating through completely in the oven to serve.

Nutritions: Calories: 178, Fat: 10g, Carbohydrates: 4g, Phosphorus: 147mg, Potassium: 272mg, Sodium: 273 Mg, Protein: 16g

128. SLOW-COOKED BEEF BRISKET

PREPARATION: 10 MIN   COOKING: 3 H 30 MIN   SERVES: 6

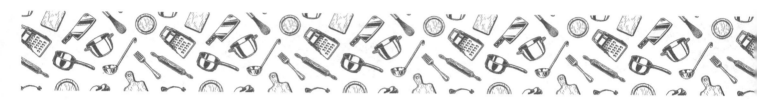

INGREDIENTS

- 10-ounce chuck roast
- 1 onion, sliced
- 1 cup carrots, peeled and sliced
- 1 tablespoon mustard
- 1 tablespoon thyme (fresh or dried)
- 1 tablespoon rosemary (fresh or dried)
- 2 garlic cloves
- 2 tablespoon extra-virgin olive oil
- 1 teaspoon black pepper
- 1 cup homemade chicken stock (p.52)
- 1 cup water

DIRECTIONS

1. Preheat the oven to 300°f/150°c/gas mark 2.
2. Trim any fat from the beef and soak vegetables in warm water.
3. Make a paste by mixing together the mustard, thyme, rosemary, and garlic, before mixing in the oil and pepper.
4. Combine this mix with the stock.
5. Pour the mixture over the beef into an oven proof baking dish.
6. Place the vegetables onto the bottom of the baking dish with the beef.
7. Cover and roast for 3 hours, or until tender.
8. Uncover the dish and to cook for 30 minutes in the oven.
9. Serve hot!

Nutritions: *Calories: 151, Fat: 7g, Carbohydrates: 7g, Phosphorus: 144mg, Potassium: 344mg, Sodium: 279mg, Protein: 15g*

129. PORK SOUVLAKI

PREPARATION: 20 MIN

COOKING: 12 MIN

SERVES: 8

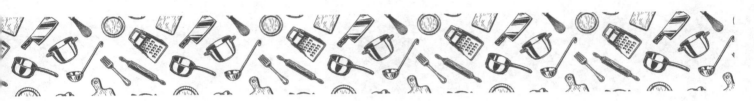

INGREDIENTS

- Olive oil – 3 tablespoons
- Lemon juice – 2 tablespoons
- Minced garlic – 1 teaspoon
- Chopped fresh oregano – 1 tablespoon
- Ground black pepper – ¼ teaspoon
- Pork leg – 1 pound, cut in 2-inch cubes

DIRECTIONS

1. In a bowl, stir together the lemon juice, olive oil, garlic, oregano, and pepper.
2. Add the pork cubes and toss to coat.
3. Place the bowl in the refrigerator, covered, for 2 hours to marinate.
4. Thread the pork chunks onto 8 wooden skewers that have been soaked in water.
5. Preheat the barbecue to medium-high heat.
6. Grill the pork skewers for about 12 minutes, turning once, until just cooked through but still juicy.

Nutritions: Calories: 95, Fat: 4g, Carb: 0g, Phosphorus: 125mg, Potassium: 230mg, Sodium: 29mg, Protein: 13g

130. OPEN-FACED BEEF STIR-UP

PREPARATION: 10 MIN

COOKING: 10 MIN

SERVES: 6

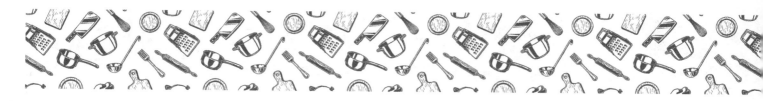

INGREDIENTS

- 95% lean ground beef – ½ pound
- Chopped sweet onion – ½ cup
- Shredded cabbage – ½ cup
- Herb pesto – ¼ cup
- Hamburger buns – 6, bottom halves only

DIRECTIONS

1. Sauté the beef and onion for 6 minutes or until beef is cooked.
2. Add the cabbage and sauté for 3 minutes more.
3. Stir in pesto and heat for 1 minute.
4. Divide the beef mixture into 6 portions and serve each on the bottom half of a hamburger bun, open-face.

Nutritions: *Calories: 120, Fat: 3g, Phosphorus: 106mg, Potassium: 198mg, Sodium: 134mg, Protein: 11g*

131. GRILLED STEAK WITH CUCUMBER SALSA

PREPARATION: 20 MIN

COOKING: 15 MIN

SERVES: 4

INGREDIENTS

For the salsa
- Chopped English cucumber - 1 cup
- Boiled and diced red bell pepper – ¼ cup
- Scallion – 1, both green and white parts, chopped
- Chopped fresh cilantro – 2 tablespoons
- Juice of 1 lime

For the steak
- Beef tenderloin steaks – 4 (3-ounce), room temperature
- Olive oil
- Freshly ground black pepper

DIRECTIONS

1. To make the salsa, in a bowl combine the lime juice, cilantro, scallion, bell pepper, and cucumber. Set aside.
2. To make the steak: preheat a barbecue to medium heat.
3. Rub the steaks with oil and season with pepper.
4. Grill the steaks for about 5 minutes per side for medium-rare, or until the desired state.
5. Serve the steaks topped with salsa.

Nutritions: *Calories: 130, Fat: 6g, Carb: 1g, Phosphorus: 186mg, Potassium: 272mg, Sodium: 39mg, Protein: 19g*

132. BEEF BRISKET

PREPARATION: 10 MIN

COOKING: 3 ½ H

SERVES: 6

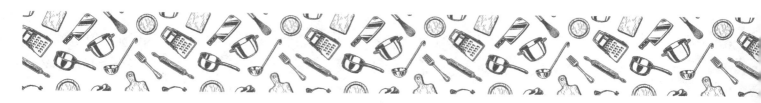

INGREDIENTS

- Chuck roast – 12 ounces trimmed
- Garlic – 2 cloves
- Thyme – 1 tablespoon
- Rosemary – tablespoon
- Mustard - 1 tablespoon
- Extra virgin olive oil – ¼ cup
- Black pepper – 1 teaspoon
- Onion – 1, diced
- Carrots – 1 cup, peeled and sliced
- Low salt stock – 2 cups

DIRECTIONS

1. Preheat the oven to 300f.
2. Soak vegetables in warm water.
3. Make a paste by mixing together the thyme, mustard, rosemary, and garlic. Then mix in the oil and pepper.
4. Add the beef to the dish.
5. Pour the mixture over the beef into a dish.
6. Place the vegetables onto the bottom of the baking dish around the beef.
7. Cover and roast for 3 hours, or until tender.
8. Uncover the dish and to cook for 30 minutes in the oven.
9. Serve.

Nutritions: Calories: 303, Fat: 25g, Carb: 7g, Phosphorus: 376mg, Potassium: 246mg, Sodium: 44mg, Protein: 18g

133. APRICOT AND LAMB TAGINE

PREPARATION: 10 MIN

COOKING: 1-1 ½ H

SERVES: 2

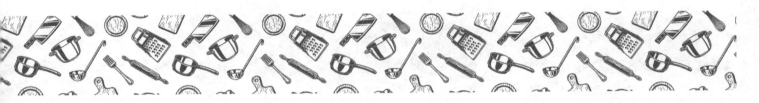

INGREDIENTS

- Extra virgin olive oil – 1 tablespoon
- Lean lamb fillets – 2, cubed
- Onion – 1, diced
- Homemade chicken stock – 4 cups
- Cumin – 1 teaspoon
- Turmeric – 1 teaspoon
- Curry powder – 1 teaspoon
- Dried rosemary – 1 teaspoon
- Chopped parsley – 1 teaspoon
- Canned apricots – ½ cup, juices drained and apricots rinsed

DIRECTIONS

1. Heat the olive oil in a pot.
2. Add lamb to the pot and cook for 5 minutes or until browned.
3. Remove lamb and set aside.
4. Add the chopped onion to the pot and sauté for 5 minutes, or until starting to soften.
5. Sprinkle with cumin, curry powder, and turmeric over the onions and continue to stir for 4 to 5 minutes.
6. Cover the pot and leave to simmer on a low heat for 1 to 1.5 hours or until the lamb is tender and fully cooked through.
7. Add the apricots 15 minutes before the end of the cooking time.
8. Garnish with parsley and serve.

Nutritions: *Calories: 193, Fat: 12g, Carb: 9g, Phosphorus: 170mg, Potassium: 156mg, Sodium: 105mg, Protein: 20g*

134. LAMB SHOULDER WITH ZUCCHINI AND EGGPLANT

PREPARATION: 10 MIN

COOKING: 4-5 H

SERVES: 2

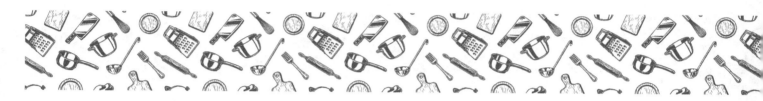

INGREDIENTS

- Lean lamb shoulder – 6 ounces
- Zucchinis – 2, cubed
- Eggplant – 1, cubed
- Black pepper – 1 teaspoon
- Extra virgin olive oil – 2 tablespoons
- Basil – 1 tablespoon
- Oregano – 1 tablespoon
- Garlic – 2 cloves, chopped

DIRECTIONS

1. Preheat the oven to its highest setting.
2. Soak the vegetables in warm water.
3. Trim any fat from the lamb shoulder.
4. Rub lamb with 1 tablespoon olive oil, pepper, and herbs.
5. Line a baking tray with the rest of the olive oil, garlic, zucchini, and eggplant.
6. Add the lamb shoulder and cover with foil.
7. Turn the oven down to 325f and add the dish into the oven.
8. Cook for 4 to 5 hours, remove and rest.
9. Slice the lamb and then serve with the vegetables.

Nutritions: Calories: 478, Fat: 31g, Carb: 13g, Phosphorus: 197mg, Potassium: 414mg, Sodium: 84mg, Protein: 33g

135. BEEF CHILI

PREPARATION: 10 MIN

COOKING: 30 MIN

SERVES: 2

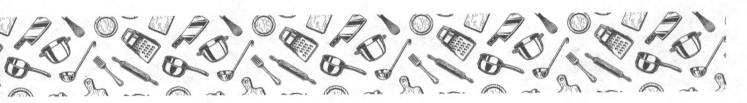

INGREDIENTS

- Onion – 1, diced
- Red bell pepper – 1, diced
- Garlic – 2 cloves, minced
- Lean ground beef – 6 ounces
- Chili powder – 1 teaspoon
- Oregano – 1 teaspoon
- Extra virgin olive oil – 2 tablespoons
- Water – 1 cup
- Brown rice -1 cup
- Fresh cilantro -1 tablespoon, to serve

DIRECTIONS

1. Soak vegetables in warm water.
2. Bring a pan of water to boil and add rice for 20 minutes.
3. Meanwhile, add the oil to a pan and heat on medium-high heat.
4. Add the pepper, onions, and garlic and sauté for 5 minutes until soft.
5. Remove and set aside.
6. Add the beef to the pan and stir until browned.
7. Add the vegetables into the pan and stir.
8. Now add the chili powder and herbs and water, cover and turn the heat down a little to simmer for 15 minutes.
9. Meanwhile, drain the water from the rice, add the lid and steam while the chili is cooking.
10. Serve hot with the fresh cilantro sprinkled over the top.

Nutritions: *Calories: 459, Fat: 22g, Carb: 36g, Phosphorus: 332mg, Potassium: 360mg, Protein: 22g*

136. SKIRT STEAK GLAZED WITH BOURBON

PREPARATION: 30 MIN

COOKING: 50 MIN

SERVES: 8

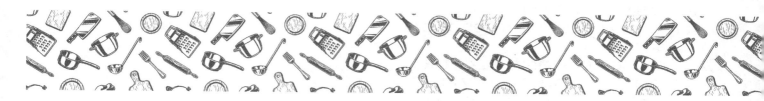

INGREDIENTS

- Bourbon glaze
- Shallots (diced) – ¼ cup
- Unsalted butter (chilled) – 3 tablespoons
- Bourbon – 1 cup
- Dark brown sugar – ¼ cup
- Dijon mustard – 2 tablespoons
- Black pepper – 1 tablespoon
- Skirt steak
- Grapeseed oil – 2 tablespoons
- Dried oregano – ½ teaspoon
- Smoked paprika – ½ teaspoon
- Black pepper – 1 teaspoon
- Red wine vinegar – 1 tablespoon
- Skirt steak – 2 pounds

DIRECTIONS

1. Start by preparing the bourbon glaze. For this, you will need to take a small saucepan and place it over a medium-high flame.
2. Add in 1 tablespoon of butter and toss in the shallots. Stir-fry until they turn brown.
3. Reduce the heat to the minimum and remove the saucepan from the stove. Pour in the bourbon and stir thoroughly. Return the saucepan to the stove.
4. Let it cook on a low flame for about 15 minutes. Make sure the glaze reduces to one-third.
5. Stir in the dark sugar, black pepper, and dijon mustard. Keep stirring until the glaze becomes bubbly.
6. Turn off the flame and add in about 2 tablespoons of cold butter. Keep stirring to incorporate with the sauce.
7. Now prepare the skirt steak. To do this, take a gallon-sized zip-lock bag and add in the grapeseed oil, dried oregano, smoked paprika, black pepper, and red wine vinegar. Mix well.

8. Now add in the steaks and shake well. Allow the steaks to sit in the marinade for about 45 minutes.
9. Remove the steaks from the zip-lock bag. Set aside.
10. Heat the grill and place the steaks on it. Cook for about 20 minutes.
11. Once done, remove the steak and place it on a baking tray. Let it rest for about 10 minutes before serving.
12. Slice the steaks and drizzle the glaze on top. Place the tray in the broiler for 5 minutes. Serve hot!

Nutritions: Protein 24g, Carbohydrates 8g, Fat 22g, Cholesterol 93mg, Sodium 152mg, Potassium 283mg, Phosphorus 171mg, Calcium 22mg, Fiber 0.5g

137. HERBY BEEF STROGANOFF AND FLUFFY RICE

PREPARATION: 15 MIN

COOKING: 5 H

SERVES: 6

INGREDIENTS

- ½ cup onion
- 2 garlic cloves
- 9ounce of flat cut beef brisket, cut into 1" cubes
- ½ cup of reduced-sodium beef stock
- 1/3 cup red wine
- ½ teaspoon dried oregano
- ¼ teaspoon freshly ground black pepper
- ½ teaspoon dried thyme
- ½ teaspoon of saffron
- ½ cup almond milk (unenriched)
- ¼ cup all-purpose flour
- 1 cup of water
- 2 ½ cups of white rice

DIRECTIONS

1. Chop the onion and mince the garlic cloves.
2. Mix the beef, stock, wine, onion, garlic, oregano, pepper, thyme and saffron in your slow cooker.
3. Cover and cook on high until the beef is tender, for about 4-5 hours.
4. Combine the almond milk, flour and water.
5. Whisk together until smooth.
6. Add the flour mixture to the slow cooker.
7. Cook for another 15 to 25 minutes until the stroganoff is thick.
8. Cook the rice using the package instructions, leaving out salt.
9. Drain off the excess water.
10. Serve the stroganoff over the rice.

Nutritions: *Calories: 241, Protein: 15g, Carbohydrates: 29g, Fat: 5g, Cholesterol: 39g, Sodium: 182mg, Potassium: 206mg, Phosphorus: 151mg, Calcium: 59mg*

138. CHUNKY BEEF AND POTATO SLOW ROAST

PREPARATION: 15 MIN

COOKING: 5-6 H

SERVES: 12

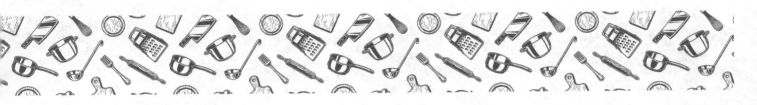

INGREDIENTS

- 3 cups of peeled potatoes, chunked
- 1 cup of onion
- 2 garlic cloves, chopped
- 1 ¼ pounds flat cut beef brisket, fat trimmed
- 2 of cups water
- 1 teaspoon of chili powder
- 1 tablespoon of dried rosemary

For the sauce:
- 1 tablespoon of freshly grated horseradish
- ½ cup of almond milk (unenriched)
- 1 tablespoon lemon juice (freshly squeezed)
- 1 garlic clove, minced
- A pinch of cayenne pepper

DIRECTIONS

1. Double boil the potatoes to reduce their potassium content.
2. (hint: bring your potato to the boil, then drain and refill with water to boil again.)
3. Chop the onion and the garlic.
4. Place the beef brisket in slow cooker.
5. Combine water, chopped garlic, chili powder and rosemary
6. Pour the mixture over the brisket.
7. Cover and cook on high for 4 hours until the meat is very tender.
8. Drain the potatoes and add them to the slow cooker.
9. Turn heat to high and cook covered until the potatoes are tender.
10. Prepare the horseradish sauce by whisking together horseradish, milk, lemon juice, minced garlic and cayenne pepper.
11. Cover and refrigerate.
12. Serve your casserole with a dash of horseradish sauce on the side.

Nutritions: Calories: 199, Protein: 21g, carbohydrates: 12g, Fat: 7g, Cholesterol: 63mg, Sodium: 282mg, Potassium: 317 Phosphorus: 191mg, calcium: 23mg, Fiber: 1g

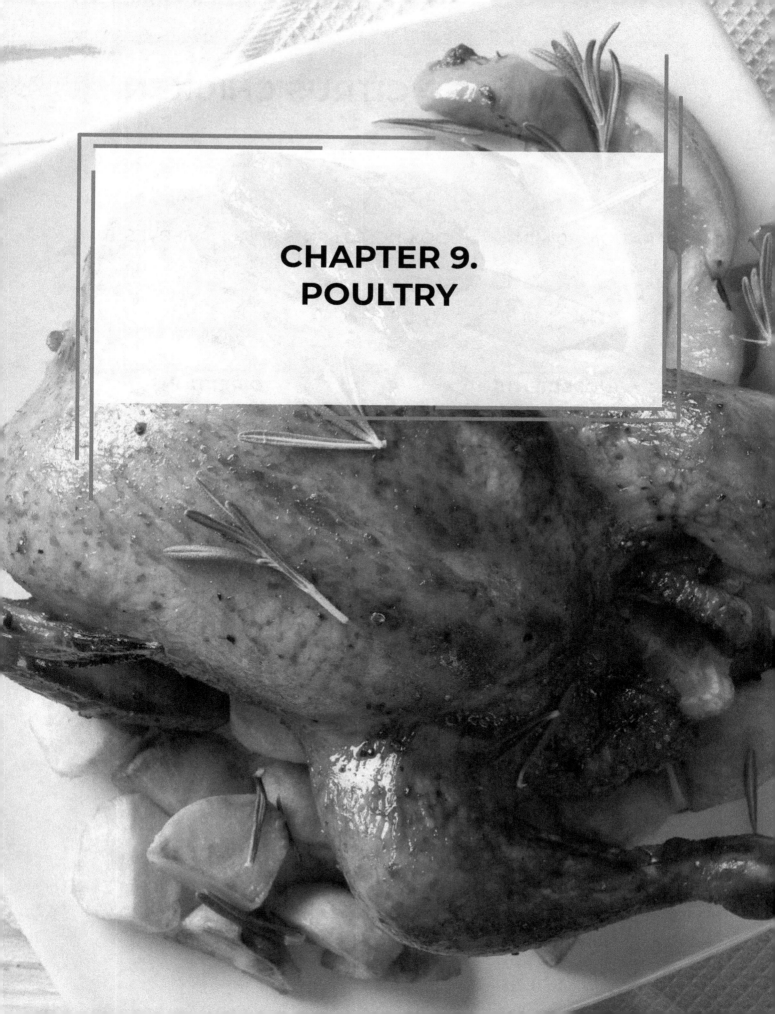

CHAPTER 9.
POULTRY

139. ROASTED CITRUS CHICKEN

PREPARATION: 20 MIN

COOKING: 60 MIN

SERVES: 8

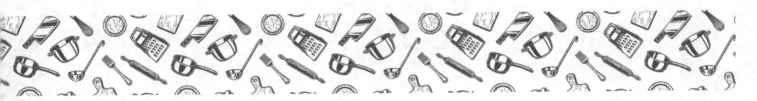

INGREDIENTS

- 1 - tablespoon olive oil
- 2 - cloves garlic, minced
- 1 - teaspoon Italian seasoning
- ½ - teaspoon black pepper
- 8 - chicken thighs
- 2 - cups chicken broth, reduced-sodium
- 3 - tablespoons lemon juice
- ½ - large chicken breast for 1 chicken thigh

DIRECTIONS

1. Warm oil in huge skillet.
2. Include garlic and seasonings.
3. Include chicken bosoms and dark-colored all sides.
4. Spot chicken in the moderate cooker and include the chicken soup.
5. Cook on low heat for 6 to 8hours
6. Include lemon juice toward the part of the bargain time.

Nutritions: *Calories: 265, Fat: 19g, Protein: 21g, Carbs: 1g*

140. CHICKEN WITH ASIAN VEGETABLES

PREPARATION: 10 MIN

COOKING: 20 MIN

SERVES: 8

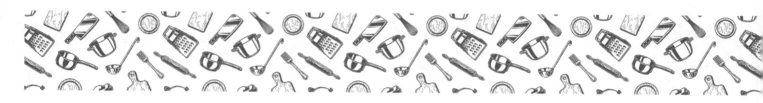

INGREDIENTS

- 2 - tablespoons canola oil
- 6 - boneless chicken breasts
- 1 - cup low-sodium chicken broth
- 3 - tablespoons reduced-sodium soy sauce
- ¼ - teaspoon crushed red pepper flakes
- 1 - garlic clove, crushed
- 1 - can (8ounces) water chestnuts, sliced and rinsed (optional)
- ½ - cup sliced green onions
- 1 - cup chopped red or green bell pepper
- 1 - cup chopped celery
- ¼ - cup cornstarch
- 1/3 - cup water
- 3 - cups cooked white rice
- ½ - large chicken breast for 1 chicken thigh

DIRECTIONS

1. Warm oil in a skillet and dark-colored chicken on all sides.
2. Add chicken to slow cooker with the remainder of the fixings aside from cornstarch and water.
3. Spread and cook on low for 6 to 8hours
4. Following 6-8 hours, independently blend cornstarch and cold water until smooth. Gradually include into the moderate cooker.
5. At that point turn on high for about 15mins until thickened. Don't close top on the moderate cooker to enable steam to leave.
6. Serve Asian blend over rice.

Nutritions: Calories: 415, Fat: 20g, Protein: 20g, Carbs: 36g

141. CHICKEN ADOBO

PREPARATION: 10 MIN

COOKING: 1 H 40 MIN

SERVES: 6

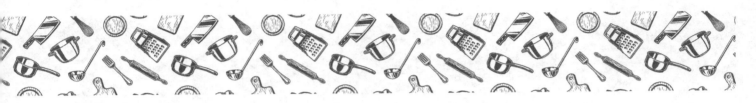

INGREDIENTS

- 4 - medium yellow onions, halved and thinly sliced
- 4 - medium garlic cloves, smashed and peeled
- 1 - (5-inch) piece fresh ginger, cut into
- 1 - inch pieces
- 1 - bay leaf
- 3 - pounds bone-in chicken thighs
- 3 - tablespoons reduced-sodium soy sauce
- ¼ - cup rice vinegar (not seasoned)
- 1 - tablespoon granulated sugar
- ½ - teaspoon freshly ground black pepper

DIRECTIONS

1. Spot the onions, garlic, ginger, and narrows leaf in an even layer in the slight cooker.
2. Take out and do away with the pores and skin from the chicken.
3. Organize the hen in an even layer over the onion mixture.
4. Whisk the soy sauce, vinegar, sugar, and pepper collectively in a medium bowl and pour it over the fowl.
5. Spread and prepare dinner on low for 8hours
6. Evacuate and take away the ginger portions and inlet leaf.
7. Present with steamed rice.

Nutritions: *Calories318, Fat: 9g, Protein: 14g, Carbs: 44g*

142. CHICKEN AND VEGGIE SOUP

PREPARATION: 15 MIN

COOKING: 25 MIN

SERVES: 8

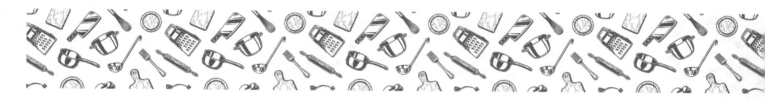

INGREDIENTS

- 4 - cups cooked and chopped chicken
- 7 - cups reduced-sodium chicken broth
- 1 - pound frozen white corn
- 1 - medium onion diced
- 4 - cloves garlic minced
- 2 - carrots peeled and diced
- 2 - celery stalks chopped
- 2 - teaspoons oregano
- 2 - teaspoon curry powder
- ½ - teaspoon black pepper

DIRECTIONS

1. Include all fixings into the moderate cooker.
2. Cook on low for 8hours
3. Serve over cooked white rice.

Nutritions: Calories220, Fat:7g, Protein: 24g, Carbs: 19g

143. TURKEY SAUSAGES

PREPARATION: 10 MIN

COOKING: 10 MIN

SERVES: 2

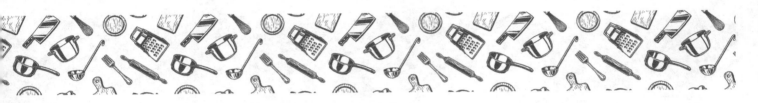

INGREDIENTS

- 1/4 teaspoon salt
- 1/8 teaspoon garlic powder
- 1/8 teaspoon onion powder
- 1 teaspoon fennel seed
- 1 pound 7% fat ground turkey

DIRECTIONS

1. Press the fennel seed and in a small cup put together turkey with fennel seed, garlic and onion powder and salt.
2. Cover the bowl and refrigerate overnight.
3. Prepare the turkey with seasoning into different portions with a circle form and press them into patties ready to be cooked.
4. Cook at a medium heat until browned.
5. Cook it for 1 to 2 minutes per side and serve them hot. Enjoy!

Nutritions: *Calories: 55, Protein: 7g, Sodium: 70mg, Potassium: 105mg, Phosphorus: 75mg*

144. ROSEMARY CHICKEN

PREPARATION: 10 MIN

COOKING: 10 MIN

SERVES: 2

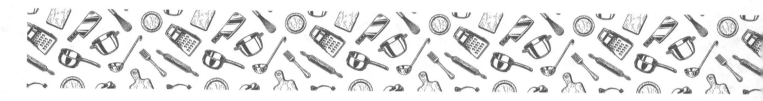

INGREDIENTS

- 2 zucchinis
- 1 carrot
- 1 teaspoon dried rosemary
- 4 chicken breasts
- 1/2 bell pepper
- 1/2 red onion
- 8 garlic cloves
- Olive oil
- 1/4 tablespoon ground pepper

DIRECTIONS

1. Prepare the oven and preheat it at 375 °f (or 200°c).
2. Slice both zucchini and carrots and add bell pepper, onion, garlic and put everything adding oil in a 13" x 9" pan.
3. Spread the pepper over everything and roast for about 10 minutes.
4. Meanwhile, lift up the chicken skin and spread black pepper and rosemary on the flesh.
5. Remove the vegetable pan from the oven and add the chicken, returning the pan to the oven for about 30 more minutes. Serve and enjoy!

Nutritions: Calories: 215 Protein: 28g Sodium: 105mg
Potassium: 580mg Phosphorus: 250mg

145. SMOKY TURKEY CHILI

PREPARATION: 5 MIN

COOKING: 45 MIN

SERVES: 8

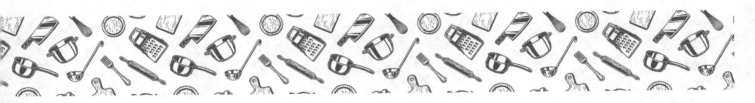

INGREDIENTS

- 12ounce lean ground turkey
- 1/2 red onion, chopped
- 2 cloves garlic, crushed and chopped
- ½ teaspoon of smoked paprika
- ½ teaspoon of chili powder
- ½ teaspoon of dried thyme
- ¼ cup reduced-sodium beef stock
- ½ cup of water
- 1 ½ cups baby spinach leaves, washed
- 3 wheat tortillas

DIRECTIONS

1. Brown the ground beef in a dry skillet over a medium-high heat.
2. Add in the red onion and garlic.
3. Sauté the onion until it goes clear.
4. Transfer the contents of the skillet to the slow cooker.
5. Add the remaining ingredients and simmer on low for 30–45 minutes.
6. Stir through the spinach for the last few minutes to wilt.
7. Slice tortillas and gently toast under the broiler until slightly crispy.
8. Serve on top of the turkey chili.

Nutritions: *Calories: 93.5, Protein: 8g, Carbohydrates: 3g, Fat: 5.5g, Cholesterol: 30.5mg, Sodium: 84.5mg, Potassium: 142.5mg, Phosphorus: 92.5mg, calcium: 29mg, Fiber: 0.5g*

146. AVOCADO-ORANGE GRILLED CHICKEN

PREPARATION: 20 MIN   **COOKING: 60 MIN**   **SERVES: 4**

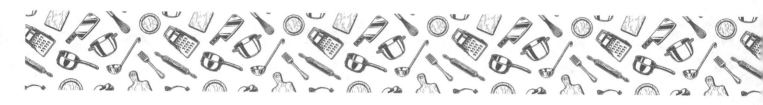

INGREDIENTS

- ¼ cup fresh lime juice
- ¼ cup minced red onion
- 1 avocado
- 1 cup low fat yogurt
- 1 small red onion, sliced thinly
- 1 tablespoon honey
- 2 oranges, peeled and sectioned
- 2 tablespoons. Chopped cilantro
- 4 pieces of 4-6ounce boneless, skinless chicken breasts
- Pepper and salt to taste

DIRECTIONS

1. In a large bowl mix honey, cilantro, minced red onion and yogurt.
2. Submerge chicken into mixture and marinate for at least 30 minutes.
3. Grease grate and preheat grill to medium high fire.
4. Remove chicken from marinade and season with pepper and salt.
5. Grill for 6 minutes per side or until chicken is cooked and juices run clear.
6. Meanwhile, peel avocado and discard seed. Chop avocados and place in bowl. Quickly add lime juice and toss avocado to coat well with juice.
7. Add cilantro, thinly sliced onions and oranges into bowl of avocado, mix well.
8. Serve grilled chicken and avocado dressing on the side.

Nutritions: Calories: 209; Carbs: 26g; Protein: 8g; Fats: 10g; Phosphorus: 157mg; Potassium: 548mg; Sodium: 125mg

147. HERBS AND LEMONY ROASTED CHICKEN

PREPARATION: 15 MIN

COOKING: 1 ½ H

SERVES: 8

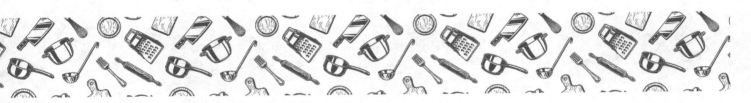

INGREDIENTS

- ½ teaspoon ground black pepper
- ½ teaspoon mustard powder
- ½ teaspoon salt
- 1 3-lb whole chicken
- 1 teaspoon garlic powder
- 2 lemons
- 2 tablespoons. Olive oil
- 2 teaspoons. Italian seasoning

DIRECTIONS

1. In small bowl, mix well black pepper, garlic powder, mustard powder, and salt.
2. Rinse chicken well and slice off giblets.
3. In a lubricated 9 x 13 baking dish, place chicken and add 1 ½ teaspoons. Of seasoning made earlier inside the chicken and rub the remaining seasoning around chicken.
4. In small bowl, mix olive oil and juice from 2 lemons. Drizzle over chicken.
5. Bake chicken in a preheated 350of oven until juices run clear, around 1 ½ hours. Every once in a while, baste chicken with its juices.

Nutritions: *Calories: 190; Carbs: 2g; Protein: 35g; Fats: 9g; Phosphorus: 341mg; Potassium: 439mg; Sodium: 328mg*

148. GROUND CHICKEN & PEAS CURRY

PREPARATION: 15 MIN

COOKING: 6-10 MIN

SERVES: 3-4

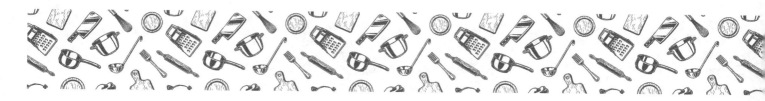

INGREDIENTS

- For marinade:
- 3 tablespoons essential olive oil
- 2 bay leaves
- 2 onions, grinded to some paste
- ½ tablespoon garlic paste
- ½ tablespoon ginger paste
- 2 tomatoes, chopped finely
- 1 tablespoon ground cumin
- 1 tablespoon ground coriander
- 1 teaspoon ground turmeric
- 1 teaspoon red chili powder
- Salt, to taste
- 1-pound lean ground chicken
- 2 cups frozen peas
- 1½ cups water
- 1-2 teaspoons garam masala powder

DIRECTIONS

1. In a deep skillet, heat oil on medium heat.
2. Add bay leaves and sauté for approximately half a minute.
3. Add onion paste and sauté for approximately 3-4 minutes.
4. Add garlic and ginger paste and sauté for around 1-1½ minutes.
5. Add tomatoes and spices and cook, stirring occasionally for about 3-4 minutes.
6. Stir in chicken and cook for about 4-5 minutes.
7. Stir in peas and water and bring to a boil on high heat.
8. Reduce the heat to low and simmer approximately 5-8 minutes or till desired doneness.
9. Stir in garam masala and remove from heat.
10. Serve hot.

Nutritions: Calories: 450, Fat: 10g, Carbohydrates: 19g, Fiber: 6g, Protein: 38g

149. CHICKEN MEATBALLS CURRY

PREPARATION: 20 MIN   **COOKING: 25 MIN**   **SERVES: 3-4**

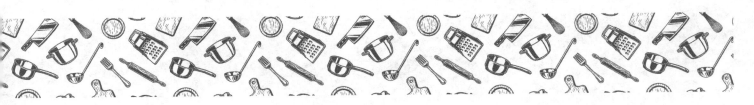

INGREDIENTS

For meatballs:
- 1-pound lean ground chicken
- 1 tablespoon onion paste
- 1 teaspoon fresh ginger paste
- 1 teaspoons garlic paste
- 1 green chili, chopped finely
- 1 tablespoon fresh cilantro leaves, chopped
- 1 teaspoon ground coriander
- ½ teaspoon cumin seeds
- ½ teaspoon red chili powder
- ½ teaspoon ground turmeric
- Salt, to taste

For curry:
- 3 tablespoons extra-virgin olive oil
- ½ teaspoon cumin seeds
- 1 (1-inch) cinnamon stick
- 3 whole cloves
- 3 whole green cardamoms
- 1 whole black cardamom
- 2 onions, chopped
- 1 teaspoon fresh ginger, minced
- 1 teaspoons garlic, minced
- 4 whole tomatoes, chopped finely
- 2 teaspoons ground coriander
- 1 teaspoon garam masala powder

DIRECTIONS

1. For meatballs in a substantial bowl, add all ingredients and mix till well combined.
2. Make small equal-sized meatballs from mixture.
3. In a big deep skillet, heat oil on medium heat.
4. Add meatballs and fry approximately 3-5 minutes or till browned from all sides.
5. Transfer the meatballs in a bowl.
6. In the same skillet, add cumin seeds, cinnamon stick, cloves, green cardamom and black cardamom and sauté approximately 1 minute.
7. Add onions and sauté for around 4-5 minutes.
8. Add ginger and garlic paste and sauté approximately 1 minute.
9. Add tomato and spices and cook, crushing with the back of spoon for approximately 2-3 minutes.
10. Add water and meatballs and provide to a boil.
11. Reduce heat to low.
12. Simmer for approximately 10 minutes.

- ½ teaspoon ground nutmeg
- ½ teaspoon red chili powder
- ½ teaspoon ground turmeric
- Salt, to taste
- 1 cup water
- Chopped fresh cilantro, for garnishing

13. Serve hot with all the garnishing of cilantro.

Nutritions: *Calories: 421, Fat: 8g, Carbohydrates: 18g, Fiber: 5g, Protein: 34g*

150. CREAMY MUSHROOM AND BROCCOLI CHICKEN

PREPARATION: 15 MIN

COOKING: 6 H

SERVES: 6

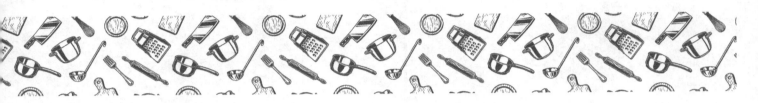

INGREDIENTS

- 1 10.5 ounce can of low-sodium cream of mushroom soup
- 1 21 ounce can of low-sodium cream of chicken soup
- 2 whole cooked chicken breasts, chopped or shredded
- 2 cup milk
- 1lb broccoli florets
- ¼ teaspoon garlic powder

DIRECTIONS

1. Place all ingredients to a 5 quart or larger slow cooker and mix well.
2. Cover and cook on low for 7 hours.
3. Serve with potatoes, pasta, or rice.

Nutritions: *Calories 155, Fat 2g, Carbs 19g, Protein 12g, Fiber 2g, Potassium 755mg, Sodium 35mg*

151. CHICKEN CURRY

PREPARATION: 10 MIN

COOKING: 4 MIN

SERVES: 4

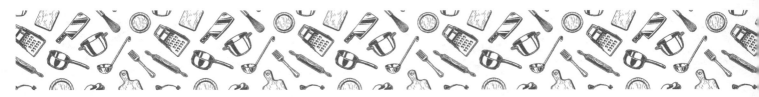

INGREDIENTS

- 1lb skinless chicken breasts
- 1 medium onion, thinly sliced
- 1 15 ounce can chickpeas, drained and rinsed well
- 2 medium sweet potatoes, peeled and diced
- ½ cup light coconut milk
- ½ cup chicken stock (see recipe)
- 1 15ounce can sodium-free tomato sauce
- 2 tablespoon curry powder
- 1 teaspoon low-sodium salt
- ½ cayenne powder
- 1 cup green peas
- 2 tablespoon lemon juice

DIRECTIONS

1. Place the chicken breasts, onion, chickpeas, and sweet potatoes into a 4 to 6-quart slow cooker.
2. Mix the coconut milk, chicken stock, tomato sauce, curry powder, salt, and cayenne together and pour into the slow cooker, stirring to coat well.
3. Cover and cook on low for 9 hours or high for 4 hours.
4. Stir in the peas and lemon juice 5 minutes before serving.

Nutritions: Calories 302, Fat 5g, Carbs 43g, Protein 24g, Fiber 9g, Potassium 573mg, Sodium 800mg

152. APPLE & CINNAMON SPICED HONEY PORK LOIN

PREPARATION: 20 MIN

COOKING: 6 H

SERVES: 6

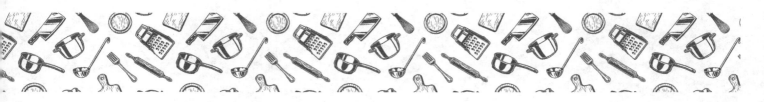

INGREDIENTS

- 1 2-3lb boneless pork loin roast
- ½ teaspoon low-sodium salt
- ¼ teaspoon pepper
- 1 tablespoon canola oil
- 3 medium apples, peeled and sliced
- ¼ cup honey
- 1 small red onion, halved and sliced
- 1 tablespoon ground cinnamon

DIRECTIONS

1. Season the pork with salt and pepper.
2. Heat oil in a skillet and brown the pork on all sides.
3. Arrange half the apples in the base of a 4 to 6-quart slow cooker.
4. Top with the honey and remaining apples.
5. Sprinkle with cinnamon and cover.
6. Cover and cook on low for 6-8 hours until the meat is tender.

Nutritions: *Calories 290, Fat 10g, Carbs 19g, Protein 29g, Fiber 2g, Potassium 789mg, Sodium 22mg*

153. LEMON & HERB TURKEY BREASTS

PREPARATION: 25 MIN

COOKING: 3 1/2 H

SERVES: 12

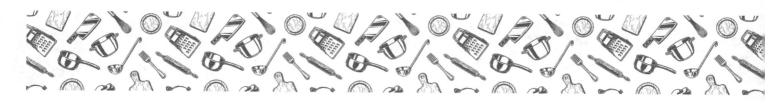

INGREDIENTS

- 1 can (14-1/2 ounces) chicken broth
- 1/2 cup lemon juice
- 1/4 cup packed brown sugar
- 1/4 cup fresh sage
- 1/4 cup fresh thyme leaves
- 1/4 cup lime juice
- 1/4 cup cider vinegar
- 1/4 cup olive oil
- 1 envelope low-sodium onion soup mix
- 2 tablespoon dijon mustard
- 1 tablespoon fresh marjoram, minced
- 1 teaspoon paprika
- 1 teaspoon garlic powder
- 1 teaspoon pepper
- ½ teaspoon low-sodium salt
- 2 2lb boneless skinless turkey breast halves

DIRECTIONS

1. Make a marinade by blending all the ingredients in a blender.
2. Pour over the turkey and leave overnight.
3. Place the turkey and marinade in a 4 to 6-quart slow cooker and cover.
4. Cover and cook on high for 3-1/2 to 4-1/2 hours or until a thermometer reads 165°.

Nutritions: Calories 219, Fat 5g, Carbs 3g, Protein 36g, Fiber 0g, Potassium 576mg, Sodium 484mg

154. CHICKEN AVOCADO SALAD

PREPARATION: 8 MIN

COOKING: 20 MIN

SERVES: 8

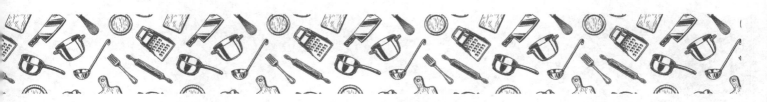

INGREDIENTS

- 3 avocados - peeled, pitted and diced
- 1-pound grilled skinless, boneless chicken breast, diced
- 1/2cupfinely chopped red onion
- 1/2cupchopped fresh cilantro
- 1/4cupbalsamic vinaigrette salad dressing

DIRECTIONS

1. Mix together the chicken, avocados, cilantro, and onion in a medium-sized bowl. Pour over the balsamic vinaigrette dressing. Toss lightly to coat all the ingredients.

Nutritions: *Calories: 252, Total Fat: 17.5g, Carbohydrates: 8.3g, Protein: 17.2g, Cholesterol: 43mg, Sodium: 130mg*

155. CHICKEN MANGO SALSA SALAD WITH CHIPOTLE LIME VINAIGRETTE

PREPARATION: 30 MIN

COOKING: 30 MIN

SERVES: 6

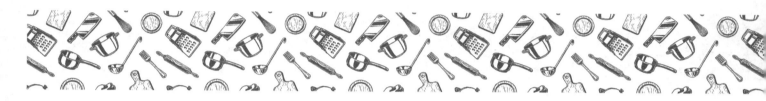

INGREDIENTS

- 1 mango - peeled, seeded and diced
- 2 roam (plum) tomatoes, chopped
- 1/2 onion, chopped
- 2 jalapeno pepper, seeded and chopped - or to taste
- 2/4cupcilantro leaves, chopped
- 1 lime, juiced
- 1/2cupolive oil
- 1/4cuplime juice
- 1/4cupwhite sugar
- 1/2 teaspoon ground chipotle chile powder
- 1/2 teaspoon ground cumin
- 1/4 teaspoon garlic powder
- 1 (10 ounce) bag baby spinach leaves
- 1cupbroccoli coleslaw mix
- 1cupdiced cooked chicken
- 3 tablespoons. Diced red bell pepper
- 3 tablespoons. Diced green bell pepper
- 2 tablespoons. Diced yellow bell pepper
- 2 tablespoons. Dried cranberries
- 2 tablespoons. Chopped pecans
- 2 tablespoons. Crumbled blue cheese

DIRECTIONS

1. In a big bowl, combine the jalapeno pepper, juiced lime, mango, cilantro, tomatoes, and onion. Set the mixture aside.
2. In a separate bowl, whisk together the garlic powder, olive oil, cumin, a quarters lime juice, chipotle, and sugar. Set the mixture aside.
3. In another big bowl, toss together the cranberries, spinach, broccoli coleslaw mix, pecans, chicken, and yellow, green and red bell peppers.
4. Top with blue cheese and mango salsa. Make sure they're spread all over.
5. Drizzle the dressing over salad. Toss to serve.

Nutritions: Calories: 317, Total Fat: 22.3g, Carbohydrates: 25g, Protein: 7.6g, Cholesterol: 14mg, Sodium: 110mg

156. CHICKEN SALAD BALSAMIC

PREPARATION: 15 MIN

COOKING: 15 MIN

SERVES: 6

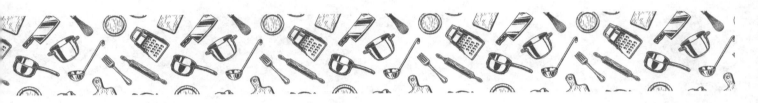

INGREDIENTS

- 3 cup diced cold, cooked chicken
- 1 cup diced apple
- 1/2 cup diced celery
- 2 green onions, chopped
- 1/2 cup chopped walnuts
- 3 tablespoons. Balsamic vinegar
- 5 tablespoons. Olive oil
- Salt and pepper to taste

DIRECTIONS

1. Toss together the celery, chicken, onion, walnuts, and apple in a big bowl.
2. Whisk the oil together with the vinegar in a small bowl. Pour the dressing over the salad. Then add pepper and salt to taste. Combine the ingredients thoroughly. Leave the mixture for 10-15 minutes. Toss once more and chill.

Nutritions: *Calories: 336, Total Fat: 26.8g, Carbohydrates: 6g, Protein: 19g, Cholesterol: 55mg, Sodium: 58mg*

157. CHICKEN SALAD WITH APPLES, GRAPES, AND WALNUTS

PREPARATION: 25 MIN   **COOKING: 25 MIN**   **SERVES: 12**

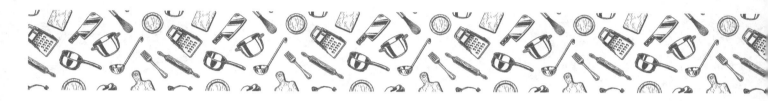

INGREDIENTS

- 4 cooked chicken breasts, shredded
- 3 granny smith apples, cut into small chunks
- 2cupchopped walnuts, or to taste
- 1/2 red onion, chopped
- 3 stalks celery, chopped
- 3 tablespoons. Lemon juice
- 1/2cupvanilla yogurt
- 5 tablespoons. Creamy salad dressing (such as miracle whip®)
- 5 tablespoons. Mayonnaise
- 25 seedless red grapes, halved

DIRECTIONS

1. In a big bowl, toss together the shredded chicken, lemon juice, apple chunks, celery, red onion, and walnuts.
2. Get another bowl and whisk together the dressing, vanilla yogurt, and mayonnaise. Pour over the chicken mixture. Toss to coat. Fold the grapes carefully into the salad.

Nutritions: Calories: 307, Total Fat: 22.7g, Carbohydrates: 10.8g, Protein: 17.3g, Cholesterol: 41mg, Sodium: 128mg

158. CHICKEN STRAWBERRY SPINACH SALAD WITH GINGER-LIME DRESSING

PREPARATION: 10 MIN

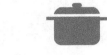

COOKING: 30 MIN

SERVES: 2

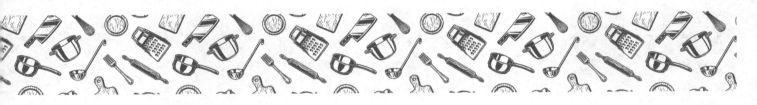

INGREDIENTS

- 2 teaspoons. Corn oil
- 1 skinless, boneless chicken breast half - cut into bite-size pieces
- 1/2 teaspoon garlic powder
- 1 1/2 tablespoons. Mayonnaise
- 1/2 lime, juiced
- 1/2 teaspoon ground ginger
- 2 teaspoons. Milk
- 2cupfresh spinach, stems removed
- 4 fresh strawberries, sliced
- 1 1/2 tablespoons. Slivered almonds
- Freshly ground black pepper to taste

DIRECTIONS

1. In a skillet, heat oil over medium heat. Add the chicken breast and garlic powder. Cook the chicken for 10 minutes per side. When the juices run clear, remove from heat and set aside.
2. Combine the lime juice, milk, mayonnaise, and ginger in a bowl.
3. Place the spinach on serving dishes. Top with strawberries and chicken. Then sprinkle with almonds. Drizzle the salad with the dressing. Add pepper and serve.

Nutritions: *Calories: 242, Total Fat: 17.3g, Carbohydrates: 7.5g, Protein: 15.8g, Cholesterol: 40mg, Sodium: 117mg*

159. ASIAN CHICKEN SATAY

PREPARATION: 15 MIN

COOKING: 10 MIN

SERVES: 6

INGREDIENTS

- Juice of 2 limes
- Brown sugar – 2 tablespoons
- Minced garlic – 1 tablespoon
- Ground cumin – 2 teaspoons
- Boneless, skinless chicken breast – 12, cut into strips

DIRECTIONS

1. In a bowl, stir together the cumin, garlic, brown sugar, and lime juice.
2. Add the chicken strips to the bowl and marinate in the refrigerator for 1 hour.
3. Heat the barbecue to medium-high.
4. Remove the chicken from the marinade and thread each strip onto wooden skewers that have been soaked in the water.
5. Grill the chicken for about 5 minutes per side or until the meat is cooked through but still juicy.

Nutritions: Calories: 78. Carb: 4g. Phosphorus: 116mg. Potassium: 108mg. Sodium: 100mg. Protein: 12g

160. ZUCCHINI AND TURKEY BURGER WITH JALAPENO PEPPERS

 PREPARATION: 15 MIN

 COOKING: 10 MIN

 SERVES: 4

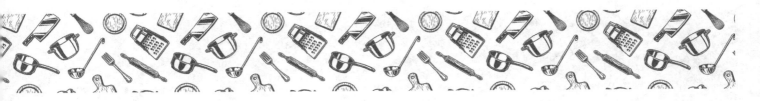

INGREDIENTS

- Turkey meat (ground) – 1 pound
- Zucchini (shredded) – 1 cup
- Onion (minced) – ½ cup
- Jalapeño pepper (seeded and minced) – 1
- Egg – 1
- Extra-spicy blend – 1 teaspoon
- Fresh poblano peppers (seeded and sliced in half lengthwise)
- Mustard – 1 teaspoon

DIRECTIONS

1. Start by taking a mixing bowl and adding in the turkey meat, zucchini, onion, jalapeño pepper, egg, and extra-spicy blend. Mix well to combine.
2. Divide the mixture into 4 equal portions. Form burger patties out of the same.
3. Prepare an electric griddle or an outdoor grill.
4. Place the burger patties on the grill and cook until the top is blistered and tender. Place the sliced poblano peppers on the grill alongside the patties. Grilling the patties should take about 5 minutes on each side.
5. Once done, place the patties onto the buns and top them with grilled peppers.

Nutritions: *Protein 25 G, Carbohydrates 5g, Fat 10g, Cholesterol 125mg, Sodium 128mg, Potassium 475 Mg, Phosphorus 280mg, Calcium 43mg, Fiber 1.6g*

161. GNOCCHI AND CHICKEN DUMPLINGS

PREPARATION: 10 MIN

COOKING: 40 MIN

SERVES: 10

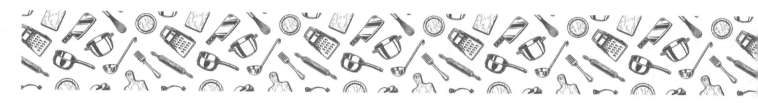

INGREDIENTS

- Chicken breast – 2 pounds
- Gnocchi – 1 pound
- Light olive oil – ¼ cup
- Better than bouillon® chicken base – 1 tablespoon
- Chicken stock (reduced-sodium) – 6 cups
- Fresh celery (diced finely) – ½ cup
- Fresh onions (diced finely) – ½ cup
- Fresh carrots (diced finely) – ½ cup
- Fresh parsley (chopped) – ¼ cup
- Black pepper – 1 teaspoon
- Italian seasoning – 1 teaspoon

DIRECTIONS

1. Start by placing the stock over a high flame. Add in the oil and let it heat through.
2. Add the chicken to the hot oil and shallow-fry until all sides turn golden brown.
3. Toss in the carrots, onions, and celery and cook for about 5 minutes. Pour in the chicken stock and let it cool on a high flame for about 30 minutes.
4. Reduce flame and add in the chicken bouillon, italian seasoning, and black pepper. Stir well.
5. Toss in the store-bought gnocchi and let it cook for about 15 minutes. Keep stirring.
6. Once done, transfer into a serving bowl. Add parsley and serve hot!

Nutritions: Protein 28g, Carbohydrates 38g, Fat 10g, Cholesterol 58mg, Sodium 121mg, Potassium 485mg, Calcium 38mg, Fiber 2g

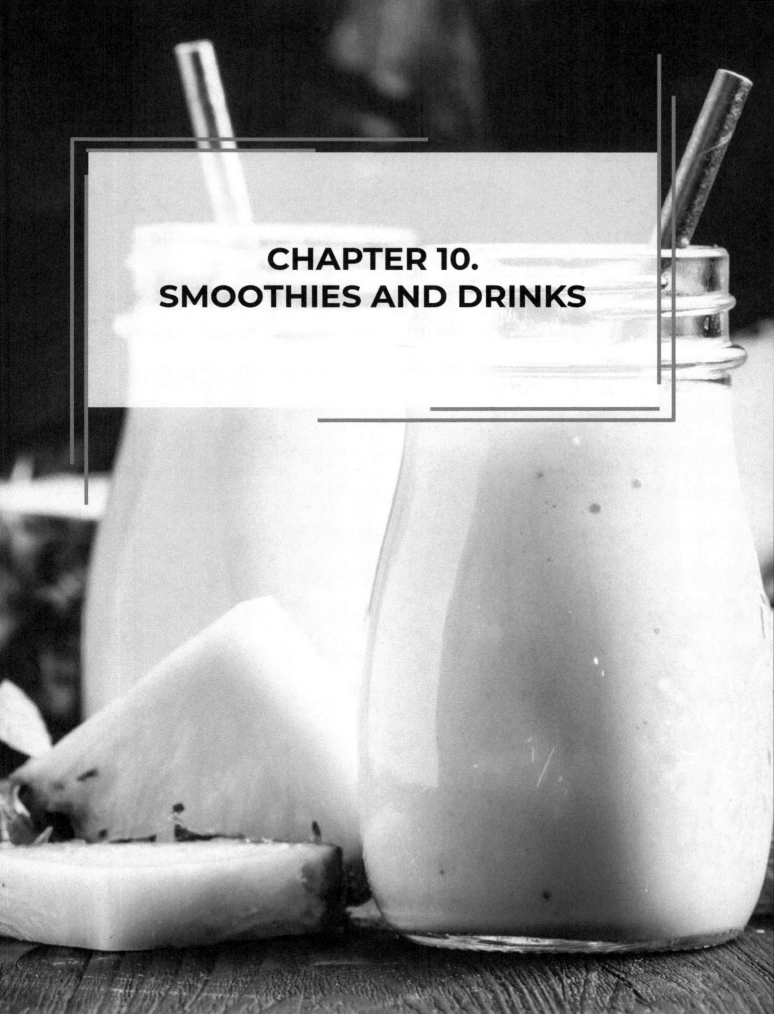

CHAPTER 10.
SMOOTHIES AND DRINKS

162. PINEAPPLE PROTEIN SMOOTHIE

PREPARATION: 10 MIN

COOKING: 0 MIN

SERVES: 1

INGREDIENTS

- 3/4 cup pineapple sorbet
- 1 scoop vanilla protein powder
- 1/2 cup water
- 2 ice cubes, optional

DIRECTIONS

1. Firstly, start by putting all the ingredients in a blender jug.
2. Give it a pulse for 30 seconds until blended well.
3. Serve chilled and fresh.

Nutritions: *Calories 268, Protein 18 g, Fat 4g, Cholesterol 36 mg, Potassium 237 mg, Calcium 160 mg, Fiber 1.4g*

163. FRUITY SMOOTHIE

PREPARATION: 10 MIN

COOKING: 0 MIN

SERVES: 2

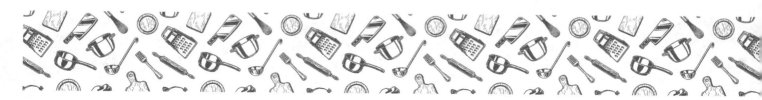

INGREDIENTS

- 8 oz canned fruits, with juice
- 2 scoops vanilla-flavored whey protein powder
- 1 cup cold water
- 1 cup crushed ice

DIRECTIONS

1. Firstly, start by putting all the ingredients in a blender jug.
2. Give it a pulse for 30 seconds until blended well.
3. Serve chilled and fresh.

Nutritions: Calories 186, Protein 23 g, Fat 2g, Cholesterol 41 mg, Potassium 282 mg, Calcium 160 mg, Fiber 1.1 g

164. MIXED BERRY PROTEIN SMOOTHIE

PREPARATION: 10 MIN

COOKING: 0 MIN

SERVES: 2

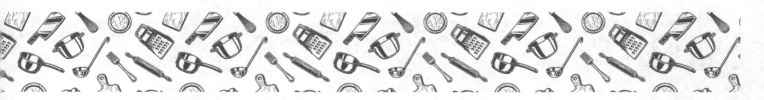

INGREDIENTS

- 4 oz cold water
- 1 cup frozen mixed berries
- 2 ice cubes
- 1 tsp blueberry essence
- 1/2 cup whipped cream topping
- 2 scoops whey protein powder

DIRECTIONS

1. Firstly, start by putting all the ingredients in a blender jug.
2. Give it a pulse for 30 seconds until blended well.
3. Serve chilled and fresh.

Nutritions: *Calories 104, Protein 6 g, Fat 4 g, Cholesterol 11 mg, Potassium 141 mg, Calcium 69 mg, Fiber 2.4 g*

165. PEACH HIGH-PROTEIN SMOOTHIE

PREPARATION: 10 MIN

COOKING: 0 MIN

SERVES: 1

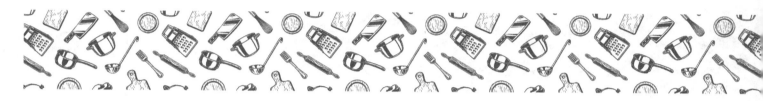

INGREDIENTS

- 1/2 cup ice
- 2 tbsp powdered egg whites
- 3/4 cup fresh peaches
- 1 tbsp sugar

DIRECTIONS

1. Firstly, start by putting all the ingredients in a blender jug.
2. Give it a pulse for 30 seconds until blended well.
3. Serve chilled and fresh.

Nutritions: Calories 132, Protein 10 g, Fat 0 g, Cholesterol 0 mg, Potassium 353 mg, Calcium 9 mg, Fiber 1.9 g

166. STRAWBERRY FRUIT SMOOTHIE

PREPARATION: 10 MIN

COOKING: 0 MIN

SERVES: 1

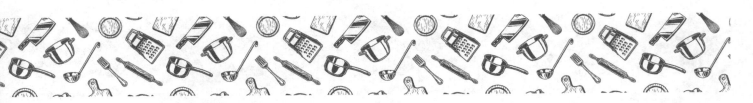

INGREDIENTS

- 3/4 cup fresh strawberries
- 1/2 cup liquid pasteurized egg whites
- 1/2 cup ice
- 1 tbsp sugar

DIRECTIONS

1. Firstly, start by putting all the ingredients in a blender jug.
2. Give it a pulse for 30 seconds until blended well.
3. Serve chilled and fresh.

Nutritions: *Calories 156, Protein 14 g, Fat 0 g, Cholesterol 0 mg, Potassium 400 mg, Phosphorus 49 mg, Calcium 29 mg, Fiber 2.5 g*

167. WATERMELON BLISS

 PREPARATION: 10 MIN

 COOKING: 0 MIN

 SERVES: 2

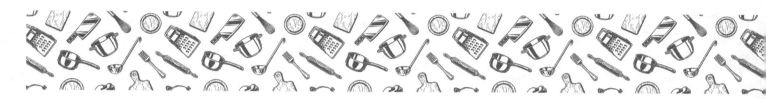

INGREDIENTS

- 2 cups watermelon
- 1 medium-sized cucumber, peeled and sliced
- 2 mint sprigs, leaves only
- 1 celery stalk
- Squeeze of lime juice

DIRECTIONS

1. Firstly, start by putting all the ingredients in a blender jug.
2. Give it a pulse for 30 seconds until blended well.
3. Serve chilled and fresh.

Nutritions: Calories 156, Protein 14 g, Fat 0 g, Cholesterol 0 mg, Potassium 400 mg, Calcium 29 mg, Fiber 2.5g

168. CRANBERRY SMOOTHIE

PREPARATION: 10 MIN

COOKING: 0 MIN

SERVES: 1

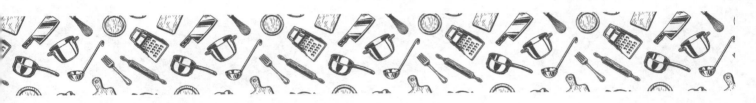

INGREDIENTS

- 1 cup frozen cranberries
- 1 medium cucumber, peeled and sliced
- 1 stalk of celery
- Handful of parsley
- Squeeze of lime juice

DIRECTIONS

1. Firstly, start by putting all the ingredients in a blender jug. Give it a pulse for 30 seconds until blended well.
2. Serve chilled and fresh.

Nutritions: *Calories 126, Protein 12 g, Fat 0.03 g, Cholesterol 0 mg, Potassium 220 mg, Calcium 19 mg, Fiber 1.4g*

169. BERRY CUCUMBER SMOOTHIE

PREPARATION: 10 MIN

COOKING: 0 MIN

SERVES: 1

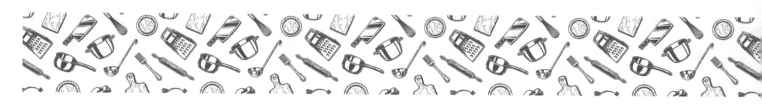

INGREDIENTS

- 1 medium cucumber, peeled and sliced
- ½ cup fresh blueberries
- ½ cup fresh or frozen strawberries
- ½ cup unsweetened rice milk
- Stevia, to taste

DIRECTIONS

1. Firstly, start by putting all the ingredients in a blender jug.
2. Give it a pulse for 30 seconds until blended well.
3. Serve chilled and fresh.

Nutritions: Calories 141, Protein 10 g, Carbohydrates 15 g, Fat 0 g, Sodium 113 mg, Potassium 230 mg, Phosphorus 129 mg

170. RASPBERRY PEACH SMOOTHIE

PREPARATION: 10 MIN

COOKING: 0 MIN

SERVES: 2

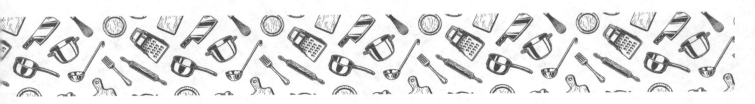

INGREDIENTS

- 1 cup frozen raspberries
- 1 medium peach, pit removed, sliced
- ½ cup silken tofu
- 1 tbsp honey
- 1 cup unsweetened vanilla almond milk

DIRECTIONS

1. Firstly, start by putting all the ingredients in a blender jug.
2. Give it a pulse for 30 seconds until blended well.
3. Serve chilled and fresh.

Nutritions: *Calories 132, Protein 9 g., Carbohydrates 14 g, Sodium 112 mg, Potassium 310 mg, Phosphorus 39 mg, Calcium 32 mg*

171. POWER-BOOSTING SMOOTHIE

PREPARATION: 5 MIN

COOKING: 0 MIN

SERVES: 2

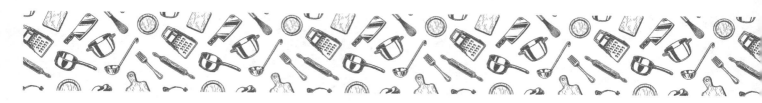

INGREDIENTS

- ½ cup water
- ½ cup non-dairy whipped topping
- 2 scoops whey protein powder
- 1½ cups frozen blueberries

DIRECTIONS

1. In a high-speed blender, add the ingredients and pulse till smooth.
2. Transfer into 2 serving glass and serve immediately.

Nutritions: Calories 242, Fat 7g, Carbs 23.8g, Protein 23.2g, Potassium (K) 263mg, Sodium (Na) 63mg, Phosphorous 30 mg

172. DISTINCTIVE PINEAPPLE SMOOTHIE

PREPARATION: 5 MIN

COOKING: 0 MIN

SERVES: 2

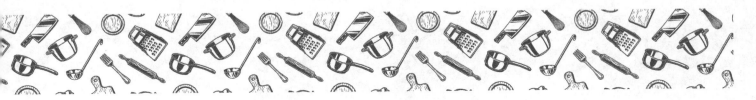

INGREDIENTS

- ¼ cup crushed ice cubes
- 2 scoops vanilla whey protein powder
- 1 cup water
- 1½ cups pineapple

DIRECTIONS

1. In a high-speed blender, add ingredients and pulse till smooth.
2. Transfer into 2 serving glass and serve immediately.

Nutritions: *Calories 117, Fat 2.1g, Carbs 18.2g, Protein 22.7g, Potassium (K) 296mg, Sodium (Na) 81mg, Phosphorous 28 mg*

173. STRENGTHENING SMOOTHIE BOWL

PREPARATION: 5 MIN

COOKING: 4 MIN

SERVES: 2

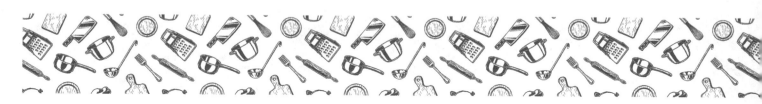

INGREDIENTS

- ¼ cup fresh blueberries
- ¼ cup fat-free plain Greek yogurt
- 1/3 cup unsweetened almond milk
- 2 tbsp of whey protein powder
- 2 cups frozen blueberries

DIRECTIONS

1. In a blender, add blueberries and pulse for about 1 minute.
2. Add almond milk, yogurt and protein powder and pulse till desired consistency.
3. Transfer the mixture into 2 bowls evenly.
4. Serve with the topping of fresh blueberries.

Nutritions: Calories 176, Fat 2.1g, Carbs 27g, Protein 15.1g, Potassium (K) 242mg, Sodium (Na) 72mg, Phosphorous 555.3 mg

174. PINEAPPLE JUICE

PREPARATION: 5 MIN

COOKING: 0 MIN

SERVES: 2

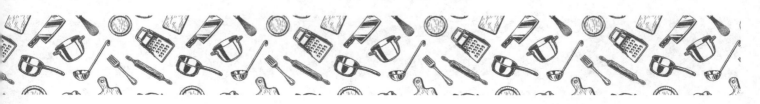

INGREDIENTS

- ½ cup canned pineapple
- 1 cup water

DIRECTIONS

1. Blend all ingredients and serve over ice.

Nutritions: *Calories 135, Protein 0 g, Carbs 0 g, Fat 0 g, Sodium (Na) 0 mg, Potassium (K) 180 mg, Phosphorus 8 mg*

175. GRAPEFRUIT SORBET

PREPARATION: 10 MIN

COOKING: 5 MIN

SERVES: 6

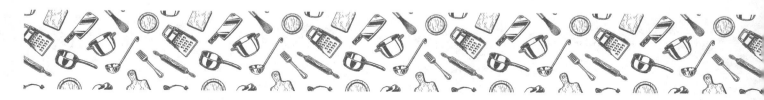

INGREDIENTS

- ½ cup sugar
- ¼ cup water
- 1 fresh thyme sprig
- For the sorbet
- Juice of 6 pink grapefruit
- ¼ cup thyme simple syrup
- To make the thyme simple syrup
- In a small saucepan, combine the sugar, water, & thyme. Bring to a boil, turn off the heat, and refrigerate, thyme sprig included, until cold. Strain the thyme sprig from the syrup.
- To make the sorbet

DIRECTIONS

1. In a blender, combine the grapefruit juice and ¼ cup of simple syrup, and process.
2. Transfer to a sealed container and freeze for 3 to 4 hours, until firm. Serve.
3. Substitution tip: Try this with other citrus fruits, such as oranges, lemons, or limes, for an equally delicious treat.

Nutritions: Calories 117, Fat 2.1g, Carbs 18.2g, Protein 22.7g, Potassium (K) 296mg, Sodium (Na) 81mg, Phosphorous 28 mg

176. APPLE AND BLUEBERRY CRISP

PREPARATION: 1 H 10 MIN

COOKING: 1 H

SERVES: 8

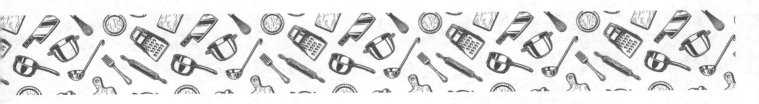

INGREDIENTS

- Crisp
- 1/4 cup of brown sugar
- 1 1/4 cups quick cooking rolled oats
- 6 tbsp non-hydrogenated melted margarine
- 1/4 cup all-purpose flour (unbleached)

Filling:
- 2 tbsp cornstarch
- 1/2 cup of brown sugar
- 2 cups chopped or grated apples
- cups frozen or fresh blueberries (not thawed)
- 1 tbsp fresh lemon juice
- 1 tbsp melted margarine

DIRECTIONS

1. Preheat the oven to 350° with the rack in the middle position.
2. Pour all the dry ingredients into a bowl, then the butter and stir until it is moistened. Set the mixture aside.
3. In an 8-inch (20-cm) square baking dish, mix the cornstarch and brown sugar. Add lemon juice and the rest of the fruits. Toss to blend the mixture. Add the crisp mixture, then bake until the crisp turns golden brown (or for 55 minutes to 1 hour). You can either serve cold or warm.

Nutritions: *Calories 127, Fat 2.1g, Carbs 18.2g, Protein 22.7g, Potassium (K) 256mgm, Sodium (Na) 61mg, Phosphorous 28 mg*

177. MINI PINEAPPLE UPSIDE DOWN CAKES

PREPARATION: 50 MIN

COOKING: 50 MIN

SERVES: 12

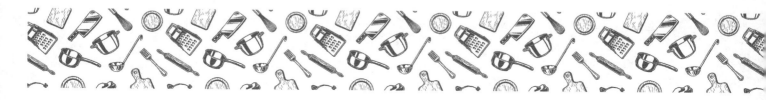

INGREDIENTS

- tbsp melted unsalted butter
- 12 canned unsweetened pineapple slices
- 1/3 cup packed brown sugar
- 2/3 cup sugar
- fresh cherries cut into halves and pitted
- tbsp canola oil
- 2/3 cup milk (fat-free)
- ½ tbsp lemon juice
- 1 large egg
- 1-1/3 cups cake flour
- 1/4 tbsp vanilla extract
- 1/4 tsp salt
- 1-1/4 tsp baking powder

DIRECTIONS

1. Coat 12 serving muffin pan with butter or you could use a square baking pan.
2. Sprinkle little brown sugar into each of the sections.
3. Crush 1 pineapple slice into each section to take the shape of the cup. Place 1 half cherry in the center of the pineapple with the cut side facing up.
4. Get a large bowl and beat the egg, milk, and the extracts until it is evenly blended.
5. Beat the flour, salt, and baking powder into sugar mixture until it is well blended to attain homogeneity and pour it into the batter prepared in the muffin pan.
6. Bake at 350°s until a toothpick sinks in and comes out clean (or for 35-40 minutes). Invert the muffin pan immediately and allow the cooked cakes to drop onto a serving plate. (If necessary, you can use a small spatula or butter knife to gently release them from the pan.)
7. Serve warm.

Nutritions: Calories 119, Fat 2.1g, Carbs 16.2g, Protein 22.7g, Potassium (K) 296mg, Sodium (Na) 81mg, Phosphorous 28 mg

178. FRESH FRUIT COMPOTE

PREPARATION: 10 MIN

COOKING: 10 MIN

SERVES: 8

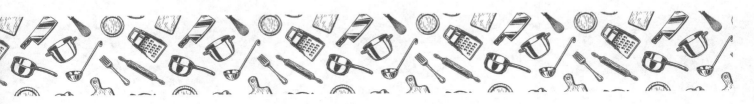

INGREDIENTS

- 1/2 cup fresh or frozen blackberries
- 1/2 cup fresh or frozen strawberries
- 1/2 cup pared peaches (diced)
- 1/2 cup fresh or frozen blueberries
- 1/2 cup orange juice (unsweetened)
- 1/4 cup frozen or fresh red raspberries (not thawed and sweetened)
- 1 banana (diced, bite-size pieces)
- 1 apple (diced, bite-size pieces)

DIRECTIONS

1. Pour some orange juice into a large container.
2. Pour all the listed ingredients.
3. Mix gently.
4. If you're using frozen fruit, let it thaw for 4 hours at ambient temperature.

Nutritions: *Calories 117, Fat 2.1g, Carbs 18.2g, Protein 22.7g, Potassium (K) 296mg, Sodium (Na) 81mg, Phosphorous 18 mg*

179. APPLE CINNAMON FARFEL KUGEL

PREPARATION: 45 MIN

COOKING: 45 MIN

SERVES: 6

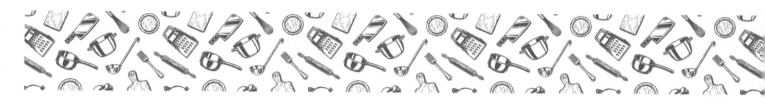

INGREDIENTS

- egg (large) whites
- 1 cup hot water
- 1/4 cup sugar
- 1 cup Matzo farfel
- 1 tbsp ground cinnamon
- 2 large apples
- 1/2 cup pineapple chunks

DIRECTIONS

1. Preheat the oven to about 375°F.
2. Peel, cut and shred the apples.
3. Get an 8" x 8" baking dish and spray it with cooking spray.
4. In another large bowl, mix the farfel and hot water.
5. Add the apples, cinnamon, and sugar.
6. Beat the egg whites and fold the egg whites.
7. Pour the drained pineapple chunks and mix together.
8. Transfer the mixture into the already prepared baking dish and sprinkle the top with additional cinnamon.
9. Bake for about 45 minutes.

Nutritions: Calories 137, Fat 2.1g, Carbs 18.2g, Protein 12.7g, Potassium (K) 296mg, Sodium (Na) 71mg, Phosphorous 28 mg

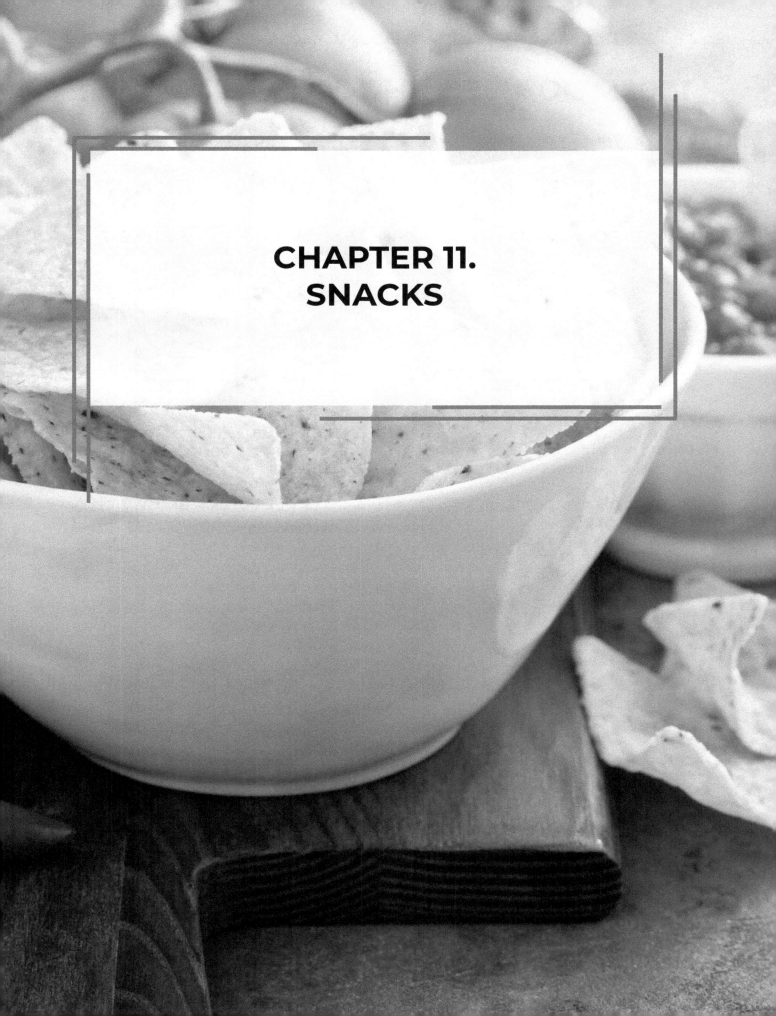

CHAPTER 11.
SNACKS

180. MOO-LESS CHOCOLATE MOUSSE

PREPARATION: 10 MIN

COOKING: 5 MIN

SERVES: 2

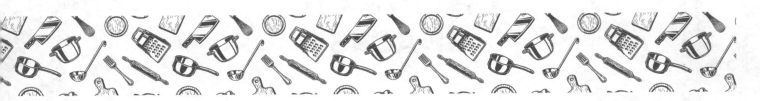

INGREDIENTS

- 2 ripe avocados
- 1 ripe banana
- 1/4 cup unsweetened cacao powder
- 2-4 tbsp coconut milk
- 1-4 tbsp maple syrup
- 1/2 tsp pure vanilla extract
- 1 pinch cinnamon
- 1 pinch sea salt

DIRECTIONS

1. Scoop out the flesh of the avocados and mash by hand.
2. Add all the ingredients in a blender and process until creamy.
3. Serve in 2 bowls. Garnish with toasted hazelnuts.

Nutritions: *Calories: 346, Carbs: 35g, Fat: 26g, Protein: 6g*

181. BAKED CARROTS

PREPARATION: 40 MIN

COOKING: 25 MIN

SERVES: 3

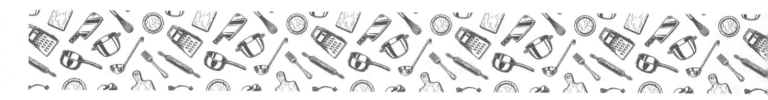

INGREDIENTS

- 1 tbsp butter;
- cloves garlic;
- Zest and juice of 1 orange;
- Handful of fresh parsley leaves;
- 1 lb carrots;
- ½ cup extra-virgin olive oil;
- 1 cup chicken stock;
- Salt and pepper to taste;

DIRECTIONS

1. Mince the garlic.
2. Slice the carrots very thinly.
3. Chop the fresh parsley leaves.
4. Mix in a bowl the garlic, orange zest and parsley.
5. Cover a roasting dish with some butter and put the previous mixture on it.
6. Arrange carrot slices on the bottom, add some olive oil on top, sprinkle with salt, pepper, garlic, zest and parsley mixture.
7. Repeat previous step until you go out of carrots.
8. Add orange juice and chicken stock.
9. Cover with a piece of wax paper. Bake for 20-25 minutes until carrots are fork-tender.

Nutritions: Calories: 109, Fat: 5.8g, Carbs: 14g, Protein: 1.4g

182. CRANBERRY & APPLE COLESLAW

PREPARATION: 15 MIN

COOKING: 10 MIN

SERVES: 6

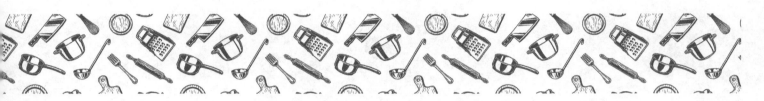

INGREDIENTS

- ½ lb cabbage;
- ½ lb shredded carrots;
- 2 granny smith apples;
- 2 cups fresh or dried cranberries;
- 1 cup mayonnaise;
- ¼ cup apple cider vinegar;
- 2 tbsp honey;

DIRECTIONS

1. Shred the cabbage and carrots.
2. Core and chop the apples in small matchsticks.
3. Combine the mayonnaise, apple cider vinegar and honey in a large bowl.
4. Add the cabbage, carrots, apples and cranberries to the bowl and mix everything together.

183. APPLE AND FENNEL SALAD

PREPARATION: 15 MIN

SERVES: 6

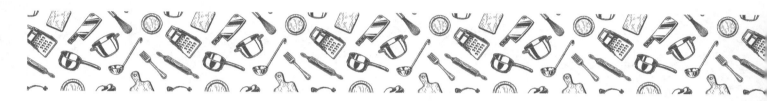

INGREDIENTS

- Ingredients:
- 1 fennel bulb;
- 1 granny smith apple;
- 2 tbsp lemon juice;
- tbsp extra-virgin olive oil;
- Fennel top;
- 1/3 tsp mustard;

DIRECTIONS

1. Slice the fennel bulb and apples.
2. Mix the mustard and lemon juice in a bowl and add the olive oil, sea salt and black pepper to taste.
3. Combine the apple and fennel slices in a bowl and pour the vinaigrette over. Add salt and pepper again.
4. Serve and garnish with the chopped fennel top.

Nutritions: Calories: 248, Fat: 10g, Carbs: 36g, Protein: 6g

184. ROASTED BEET & CANNED SARDINE SALAD

PREPARATION: 10 MIN

COOKING: 2 H

SERVES: 4

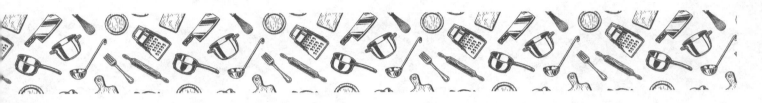

INGREDIENTS

- ½ cup mayonnaise;
- 1 tbsp prepared horseradish;
- 2 tbsp fresh dill;
- 1 lb beets, stems trimmed;
- 2 cans sardine;
- Butter;
- Salt and pepper to taste;

DIRECTIONS

1. Chop the fresh dill.
2. Clean the beets and place them individually in small closed-up foil packets.
3. Place them in a roasting dish and roast for about 45 minutes to an hour, until a fork enters the flesh easily. Put on a plate to cool.
4. When cool enough to handle, cut the beets into ½-inch cubes and place in a bowl with 2 tbsp butter. Toss well to coat the beets all over with the fat.
5. Mix the mayonnaise, dill and horseradish in a bowl and add salt and pepper to taste.
6. Place a bed of roasted beets on each plate and add the mayonnaise on top. Place the sardines on top of the mayonnaise.

Nutritions: *Calories: 393, Fat: 23.2g, Carbs: 33.5g, Protein: 17.4g*

185. CHICKEN & ZUCCHINI HOT SALAD

PREPARATION: 40 MIN   COOKING: 15 MIN   SERVES: 4

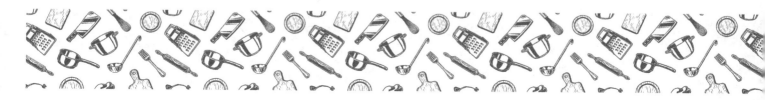

INGREDIENTS

- 2 ½ lbs chicken breasts;
- zucchinis;
- tbsp butter;
- 1 tbsp oregano;
- 1 large onion;
- tbsp mayonnaise;
- Juice of 2 lemons;
- 2 cloves garlic;
- Salt and pepper to taste;

DIRECTIONS

1. Cut the chicken breasts and zucchinis into cubes.
2. Mince the garlic and chop the onion.
3. Heat a big frying pan over a medium-high heat, add some butter and cook the chicken cubes and until well cooked. Put on a plate.
4. Add the onion to the same pan and cook about 5 minutes. Add the zucchini cubes, oregano, salt and pepper to taste. Cook until soft. Blend the mayonnaise, lemon juice and garlic in a bowl.
5. Add the cooked chicken, onion and zucchini to the sauce and mix well. You may add some lettuce onion.

Nutritions: Calories: 76, Fat: 3.8g, Carbs: 10.5g, Protein: 1.8g

186. TUNA SALAD

PREPARATION: 10 MIN

COOKING: 2 MIN

SERVES: 2

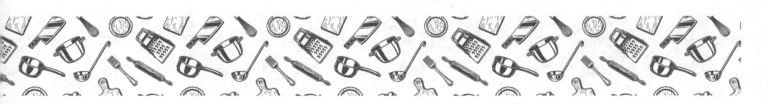

INGREDIENTS

- 2 can (12 oz) tuna;
- tsp mayonnaise;
- 2 tsp pickle relish (naturally fermented);
- 2 tsp mustard;
- 2 celery stalks;
- ½ cup onion;
- Pepper to taste;

DIRECTIONS

1. Chop the stalks and onion.
2. Mix everything together in a bowl, adjusting the texture and taste with more or less mustard and mayonnaise.
3. Add only pepper because the canned tuna is salted already

Nutritions: *Calories: 51, Fat: 1g, Carb: 9g, Phosphorus: 19mg, Potassium: 14mg, Sodium: 102mg, Protein: 1g*

187. GINGER-LIME GRILLED SHRIMP

PREPARATION: 5 MIN

COOKING: 6 MIN

SERVES: 3-4

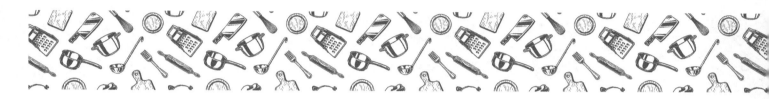

INGREDIENTS

- 2 tbsp lime juice;
- ¼ tbsp crushed red pepper flakes;
- cloves garlic;
- 2 tsp freshly-grated ginger;
- ¼ tsp salt;
- ¼ tsp ground black pepper;
- 2 tbsp fresh cilantro leaves;
- 1 tbsp extra-virgin olive oil;
- 1-2 pounds large shrimp;

DIRECTIONS

1. Mince the garlic and cilantro leaves.
2. Mix lime juice, red pepper flakes, garlic, ginger, salt, black pepper, and cilantro in a bowl, and then drizzle in the oil, stirring constantly.
3. Pierce the shrimp at the head and carefully cut along the back toward the tail, removing the dark vein.
4. Rinse in running water. Pat dry, and then place in a bowl and mix with the
5. Marinade well. Cover tightly and place into the fridge for 20 minutes.
6. Preheat the gas grill on high heat.
7. Thread the shrimp on skewers, leaving a little room among them. Grill for 2-3 minutes per side with the lid closed.

Nutritions: Calories: 23.5, Fat: 13g, Carbs: 0.6g, Protein: 2g

188. SEAFOOD JAMBALAYA

PREPARATION: 20 MIN

COOKING: 25 MIN

SERVES: 4

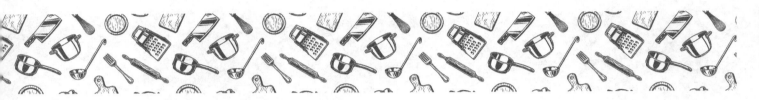

INGREDIENTS

- 1 lb wild Alaskan cod fillets;
- 1 lb shrimp;
- 2 cups chicken broth;
- 2 red bell peppers;
- 4-5 carrots;
- 1 leek;
- Sea salt to taste;
- 1 tbsp chili powder;
- ½ tsp paprika;
- ½ tsp black pepper;
- cloves garlic;
- ¼ cup organic butter;
- Hot sauce to taste;

DIRECTIONS

1. Remove shrimp's tails and shells.
2. Slice the peppers and carrots. Dice leek, mince garlic.
3. Pat the fish and shrimp dry with a paper towel.
4. Cut the fish into medium pieces.
5. Melt the butter in a large soup pot, add carrots and stew for 4 minutes.
6. Add the bell peppers and garlic and cook for another 3-4 minutes.
7. Add all the spices and the chicken broth and bring to a boil.
8. Then add the fish and shrimp and simmer until the fish begins to flake and the shrimp turn pink and float.
9. Add the hot sauce and stir well.

Nutritions: *Calories: 207.6, Fat: 4.4g, Carbs: 30.1g, Protein: 11.6g*

189. KALE CHIPS

PREPARATION: 20 MIN

COOKING: 25 MIN

SERVES: 6

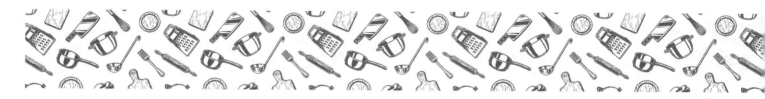

INGREDIENTS

- 2 cups Kale
- 2 tsp of olive oil
- ¼ tsp of chili powder
- Pinch cayenne pepper

DIRECTIONS

1. Preheat the oven to 300F.
2. Line 2 baking sheets with parchment paper.
3. Remove the stems from the kale and tear the leaves into 2-inch pieces.
4. Wash the kale and dry it completely.
5. Transfer the kale to a large bowl and drizzle with olive oil.
6. Use your hands to toss the kale with oil, taking care to coat each leaf evenly.
7. Season the kale with chili powder and cayenne pepper and toss to combine thoroughly.
8. Spread the seasoned kale in a single layer on each baking sheet. Do not overlap the leaves.
9. Bake the kale, rotating the pans once, for 20 to 25 minutes until it is crisp and dry.
10. Remove the trays from oven and allow the chips to cool on the trays for 5 minutes.
11. Serve.

Nutritions: Calories: 24, Fat: 2g, Carb: 2g, Phosphorus: 21mg, Potassium: 111mg, Sodium: 13mg, Protein: 1g

190. TORTILLA CHIPS

PREPARATION: 15 MIN

COOKING: 10 MIN

SERVES: 6

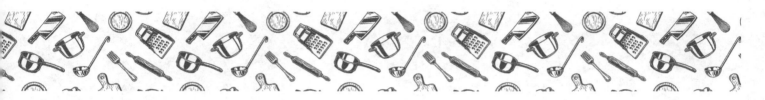

INGREDIENTS

- 2 tsp granulated sugar
- ½ tsp ground cinnamon
- Pinch ground nutmeg
- Flour tortillas – 3 (6-inch)
- Cooking spray

DIRECTIONS

1. Preheat the oven to 350F.
2. Line a baking sheet with parchment paper.
3. In a bowl, stir together the sugar, cinnamon, and nutmeg.
4. Lay the tortillas on a clean work surface and spray both sides of each lightly with cooking spray.
5. Sprinkle the cinnamon sugar evenly over both sides of each tortilla.
6. Cut the tortillas into 16 wedges each and place them on the baking sheet.
7. Bake the tortilla wedges, turning once, for about 10 minutes or until crisp.
8. Cool the chips serve.

Nutritions: *Calories: 51, Fat: 1g, Carb: 9g, Phosphorus: 29mg, Potassium: 24mg, Sodium: 103mg, Protein: 1g*

191. BUFFALO CAULIFLOWER BITES WITH DAIRY FREE RANCH DRESSING

PREPARATION: 15 MIN

COOKING: 30 MIN

SERVES: 8

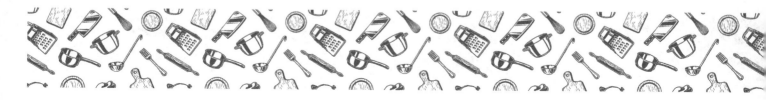

INGREDIENTS

- cups of cauliflower florets
- 2 tablespoons of extra virgin olive oil
- ¼ teaspoon of salt
- ¼ teaspoon of smoked paprika
- ¼ teaspoon of garlic powder
- ½ cup of sugar free hot sauce I used Archie Moore's brand
- Dairy Free Ranch Dressing
- 1 cup organic mayonnaise
- ½ cup of Silk unsweetened coconut milk
- 1 teaspoon of garlic powder
- 1 teaspoon of onion powder
- ¼ teaspoon of pepper
- 1 tablespoon of fresh lemon juice
- ¼ cup fresh chopped parsley
- Get Ingredients Powered by Chicory

DIRECTIONS

1. First heat oven to 400 degrees F.
2. Spray the baking sheet with nonstick olive oil cooking spray.
3. Place florets in a large bowl and toss with olive oil.
4. In a small bowl mix the salt, paprika and garlic powder together with hot sauce.
5. Add the hot sauce into cauliflower bowl and stir well until well coated. Spread the cauliflower out evenly on baking sheet and bake for 30 minutes.
6. Whisk ingredients together and pour into a mason jar. Cover and refrigerate until ready to serve with cauli bites.

Nutritions: Calories: 123, Fat: 16g, Carbohydrates: 12g, Fiber: 3g, Protein: 39g

192. BAKED CREAM CHEESE CRAB DIP

PREPARATION: 5 MIN

COOKING: 30 MIN

SERVES: 12

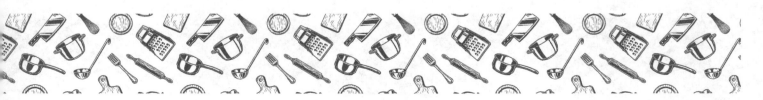

INGREDIENTS

- oz. lump crab meat
- oz. cream cheese softened
- ½ cup avocado mayonnaise
- 1 tablespoon lemon juice
- 1 teaspoon Worcestershire sauce
- ½ teaspoon of garlic powder
- ½ teaspoon of onion powder
- ½ teaspoon of salt
- ¼ teaspoon of dry mustard
- ¼ teaspoon of black pepper

DIRECTIONS

1. Add all the ingredients into small baking dish and spread out evenly.
2. Bake at 375°F for about 25 to 30 minutes.
3. Serve with low carb crackers or vegetables. Enjoy.

Nutritions: *Calories: 167, Fat: 12g,, Carbohydrates: 21g, Fiber: 2g, Protein: 31g*

193. FLUFFY MOCK PANCAKES

PREPARATION: 5 MIN

COOKING: 10 MIN

SERVES: 2

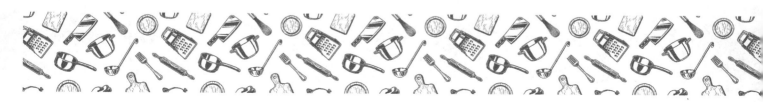

INGREDIENTS

- 1 egg
- 1 cup ricotta cheese
- 1 teaspoon cinnamon
- 2 tablespoons honey, add more if needed

DIRECTIONS

1. Using a blender, put together egg, honey, cinnamon, and ricotta cheese. Process until all ingredients are well combined.
2. Pour an equal amount of the blended mixture into the pan. Cook each pancake for 4 minutes on both sides. Serve.

Nutritions: Calories: 188.1kcal, Total Fat: 14.5g, Saturated Fat: 4.5g, Cholesterol: 139.5mg, Sodium: 175.5mg, Total Carbs: 5.5g, Fiber: 2.8g, Sugar: 0.9g, Protein: 8.5g

194. MIXES OF SNACK

PREPARATION: 10 MIN

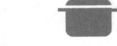

COOKING: 1 H 15 MIN

SERVES: 4

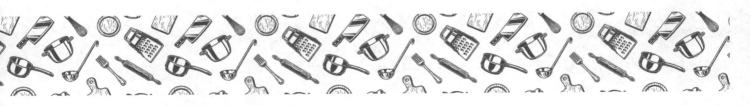

INGREDIENTS

- 6 cup margarine
- 2 tablespoon Worcestershire sauce
- 1 ½ tablespoon spice salt
- ¾ cup garlic powder
- ½ teaspoon onion powder
- 3 cups crispi
- 3 cups cheerios
- 3 cups corn flakes
- 1 cup kixe
- 1 cup pretzels
- 1 cup broken bagel chips into 1-inch pieces

DIRECTIONS

1. Preheat the oven to 250f (120c)
2. Melt the margarine in a pan. Stir in the seasoning. Gradually add the ingredients remaining by mixing so that the coating is uniform.
3. Cook 1 hour, stirring every 15 minutes. Spread on paper towels to let cool. Store in a tightly-closed container.

Nutritions: *Calories: 200kcal, Total Fat: 9g, Saturated Fat: 3.5g, Cholesterol: 0mg, Sodium: 3.5mg, Total Carbs: 27g, Fiber: 2g, Sugar: 0g, Protein: 3g*

195. CRANBERRY DIP WITH FRESH FRUIT

PREPARATION: 10 MIN

COOKING: 0 MIN

SERVES: 8

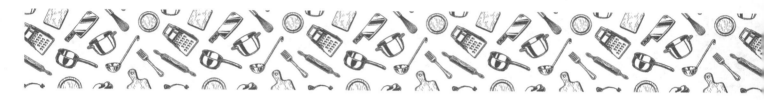

INGREDIENTS

- 8-ounce sour cream
- 1/2 cup whole berry cranberry sauce
- 1/4 teaspoon nutmeg
- 1/4 teaspoon ground ginger
- 4 cups fresh pineapple, peeled, cubed
- 4 medium apples, peeled, cored and cubed
- 4 medium pears, peeled, cored and cubed
- 1 teaspoon lemon juice

DIRECTIONS

1. Start by adding cranberry sauce, sour cream, ginger, and nutmeg to a food processor.
2. Blend the mixture until its smooth then transfer it to a bowl.
3. Toss the pineapple, with pears, apples, and lemon juice in a salad bowl.
4. Thread the fruits onto mini skewers.
5. Serve them with the sauce.

Nutritions: Calories 70. Protein 0 g. Carbohydrates 13 g. Fat 2 g. Cholesterol 4 mg. Sodium 8 mg. Potassium 101 mg. Phosphorus 15 mg. Calcium 17 mg. Fiber 1.5 g.

196. CUCUMBERS WITH SOUR CREAM

PREPARATION: 10 MIN

COOKING: 0 MIN

SERVES: 4

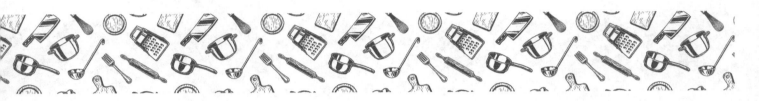

INGREDIENTS

- 2 medium cucumbers, peeled and sliced thinly
- 1/2 medium sweet onion, sliced
- 1/4 cup white wine vinegar
- 1 tablespoon canola oil
- 1/8 teaspoon black pepper
- 1/2 cup reduced-fat sour cream

DIRECTIONS

1. Toss in cucumber, onion, and all other ingredients in a medium-size bowl.
2. Mix well and refrigerate for 2 hours.
3. Toss again and serve to enjoy.

Nutritions: *Calories 64. Protein 1 g. Carbohydrates 4 g. Fat 5 g. Cholesterol 3 mg. Sodium 72 mg. Potassium 113 mg. Phosphorus 24 mg. Calcium 21 mg. Fiber 0.8 g.*

197. SWEET SAVORY MEATBALLS

PREPARATION: 10 MIN

COOKING: 20 MIN

SERVES: 12

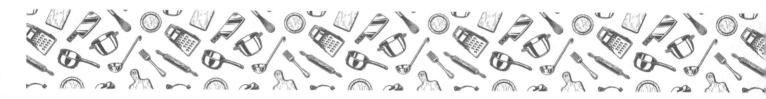

INGREDIENTS

- 1-pound ground turkey
- 1 large egg
- 1/4 cup bread crumbs
- 2 tablespoon onion, finely chopped
- 1 teaspoon garlic powder
- 1/2 teaspoon black pepper
- 1/4 cup canola oil
- 6-ounce grape jelly
- 1/4 cup chili sauce

DIRECTIONS

1. Place all ingredients except chili sauce and jelly in a large mixing bowl.
2. Mix well until evenly mixed then make small balls out of this mixture.
3. It will make about 48 meatballs. Spread them out on a greased pan on a stovetop.
4. Cook them over medium heat until brown on all the sides.
5. Mix chili sauce with jelly in a microwave-safe bowl and heat it for 2 minutes in the microwave.
6. Pour this chili sauce mixture onto the meatballs in the pan.
7. Transfer the meatballs in the pan to the preheated oven.
8. Bake the meatballs for 20 minutes in an oven at 375 degrees f.
9. Serve fresh and warm.

Nutritions: Calories 127. Protein 9 g. Carbohydrates 14 g. Fat 4 g. Cholesterol 41 mg. Sodium 129 mg. Potassium 148 mg. Phosphorus 89 mg. Calcium 15 mg. Fiber 0.2 g.

198. SPICY CORN BREAD

PREPARATION: 10 MIN **COOKING: 30 MIN** **SERVES: 8**

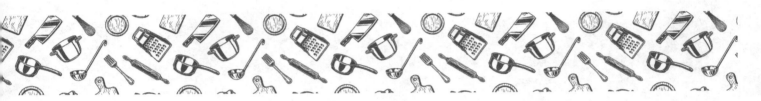

INGREDIENTS

- 1 cup all-purpose white flour
- 1 cup plain cornmeal
- 1 tablespoon sugar
- 2 teaspoon baking powder
- 1 teaspoon chili powder
- 1/4 teaspoon black pepper
- 1 cup rice milk, unenriched
- 1 egg
- 1 egg white
- 2 tablespoon canola oil
- 1/2 cup scallions, finely chopped
- 1/4 cup carrots, finely grated
- 1 garlic clove, minced

DIRECTIONS

1. Preheat your oven to 400 degrees f.
2. Now start by mixing the flour with baking powder, sugar, cornmeal, pepper and chili powder in a mixing bowl.
3. Stir in oil, milk, egg white, and egg.
4. Mix well until it's smooth then stir in carrots, garlic, and scallions.
5. Stir well then spread the batter in an 8-inch baking pan greased with cooking spray.
6. Bake for 30 minutes until golden brown.
7. Slice and serve fresh.

Nutritions: *Calories 188. Protein 5 g. Carbohydrates 31 g. Fat 5 g. Cholesterol 26 mg. Sodium 155 mg. Potassium 100 mg. Phosphorus 81 mg. Calcium 84 mg. Fiber 2 g.*

199. SWEET AND SPICY TORTILLA CHIPS

PREPARATION: 10 MIN

COOKING: 8 MIN

SERVES: 6

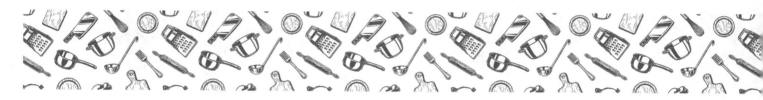

INGREDIENTS

- 1/4 cup butter
- 1 teaspoon brown sugar
- 1/2 teaspoon ground chili powder
- 1/2 teaspoon garlic powder
- 1/2 teaspoon ground cumin
- 1/4 teaspoon ground cayenne pepper
- 6 flour tortillas, 6" size

DIRECTIONS

1. Preheat oven to 425 degrees f.
2. Grease a baking sheet with cooking spray.
3. Add all spices, brown sugar, and melted butter to a small bowl.
4. Mix well and set this mixture aside.
5. Slice the tortillas into 8 wedges and brush them with the sugar mixture.
6. Spread them on the baking sheet and bake them for 8 minutes.
7. Serve fresh.

Nutritions: Calories 115. Protein 2 g. Carbohydrates 11 g. Fat 7 g. Cholesterol 15 mg. Sodium 156 mg. Potassium 42 mg. Phosphorus 44 mg. Calcium 31 mg. Fiber 0.6 g.

200. ADDICTIVE PRETZELS

PREPARATION: 10 MIN

COOKING: 1 H

SERVES: 6

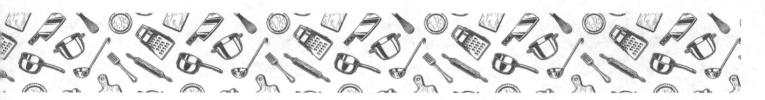

INGREDIENTS

- 32-ounce bag unsalted pretzels
- 1 cup canola oil
- 2 tablespoon seasoning mix
- 3 teaspoon garlic powder
- 3 teaspoon dried dill weed

DIRECTIONS

1. Preheat oven to 175 degrees f.
2. Place the pretzels on a cooking sheet and break them into pieces.
3. Mix garlic powder and dill in a bowl and reserve half of the mixture.
4. Mix the remaining half with seasoning mix and ¾ cup of canola oil.
5. Pour this oil over the pretzels and brush them liberally
6. Bake the pieces for 1 hour then flip them to bake for another 15 minutes.
7. Allow them to cool then sprinkle the remaining dill mixture and drizzle more oil on top.
8. Serve fresh and warm.

Nutritions: *Calories 184. Protein 2 g. Carbohydrates 22 g. Fat 8 g. Cholesterol 0 mg. Sodium 60 mg. Potassium 43 mg. Phosphorus 28 mg. Calcium 2 mg. Fiber 1.0 g.*

201. SHRIMP SPREAD WITH CRACKERS

PREPARATION: 10 MIN

COOKING: 0 MIN

SERVES: 6

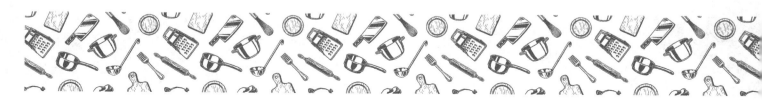

INGREDIENTS

- 1/4 cup light cream cheese
- 2 1/2-ounce cooked, shelled shrimp, minced
- 1 tablespoon no-salt-added ketchup
- 1/4 teaspoon hot sauce
- 1 teaspoon worcestershire sauce
- 1/2 teaspoon herb seasoning blend
- 24 matzo cracker miniatures
- 1 tablespoon parsley

DIRECTIONS

1. Start by tossing the minced shrimp with cream cheese in a bowl.
2. Stir in worcestershire sauce, hot sauce, herb seasoning, and ketchup.
3. Mix well and garnish with minced parsley.
4. Serve the spread with the crackers.

Nutritions: Calories 57. Protein 3 g. Carbohydrates 7 g. Fat 1 g. Cholesterol 21 mg. Sodium 69 mg. Potassium 54 mg. Phosphorus 30 mg. Calcium 15 mg. Fiber 0.2 g.

202. BUFFALO CHICKEN DIP

PREPARATION: 10 MIN

COOKING: 3 H

SERVES: 4

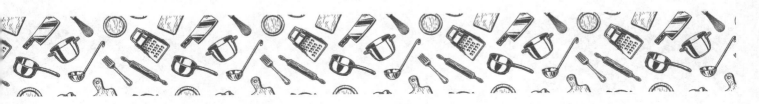

INGREDIENTS

- 4-ounce cream cheese
- 1/2 cup bottled roasted red peppers
- 1 cup reduced-fat sour cream
- 4 teaspoon hot pepper sauce
- 2 cups cooked, shredded chicken

DIRECTIONS

1. Blend half cup of drained red peppers in a food processor until smooth.
2. Now, thoroughly mix cream cheese, and sour cream with the pureed peppers in a bowl.
3. Stir in shredded chicken and hot sauce then transfer the mixture to a slow cooker.
4. Cook for 3 hours on low heat.
5. Serve warm with celery, carrots, cauliflower, and cucumber.

Nutritions: *Calories 73. Protein 5 g. Carbohydrates 2 g. Fat 5 g. Cholesterol 25 mg. Sodium 66 mg. Potassium 81 mg. Phosphorus 47 mg. Calcium 31 mg. Fiber 0 g.*

203. CHICKEN PEPPER BACON WRAPS

PREPARATION: 10 MIN

COOKING: 15 MIN

SERVES: 4

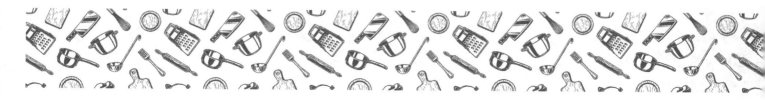

INGREDIENTS

- 1 medium onion, chopped
- 12 strips bacon, halved
- 12 fresh jalapenos peppers
- 12 fresh banana peppers
- 2 pounds boneless, skinless chicken breast

DIRECTIONS

1. Grease a grill rack with cooking spray and preheat the grill on low heat.
2. Slice the peppers in half lengthwise then remove their seeds.
3. Dice the chicken into small pieces and divide them into each pepper.
4. Now spread the chopped onion over the chicken in the peppers.
5. Wrap the bacon strips around the stuffed peppers.
6. Place these wrapped peppers in the grill and cook them for 15 minutes.
7. Serve fresh and warm.

Nutritions: Calories 71. Protein 10 g. Carbohydrates 1 g. Fat 3 g. Cholesterol 26 mg. Sodium 96 mg. Potassium 147 mg. Phosphorus 84 mg. Calcium 9 mg. Fiber 0.8 g.

204. GARLIC OYSTER CRACKERS

PREPARATION: 10 MIN

COOKING: 45 MIN

SERVES: 4

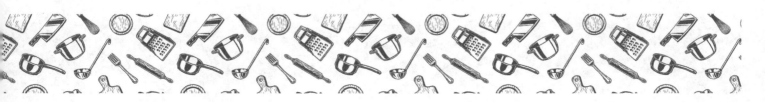

INGREDIENTS

- 1/2 cup butter-flavored popcorn oil
- 1 tablespoon garlic powder
- 7 cups oyster crackers
- 2 teaspoon dried dill weed

DIRECTIONS

1. How to prepare:
2. Preheat oven to 250 degrees f.
3. Mix garlic powder with oil in a large bowl.
4. Toss in crackers and mix well to coat evenly.
5. Sprinkle the dill weed over the crackers and toss well again.
6. Spread the crackers on the baking sheet and bake them for 45 minutes.
7. Toss them every 15 minutes.
8. Serve fresh.

Nutritions: *Calories 118. Protein 2 g. Carbohydrates 12 g. Fat 7 g. Cholesterol 0 mg. Sodium 166 mg. Potassium 21 mg. Phosphorus 15 mg. Calcium 4 mg. Fiber 3 g.*

205. LIME CILANTRO RICE

PREPARATION: 5 MIN

COOKING: 20 MIN

SERVES: 2

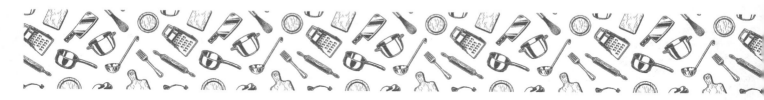

INGREDIENTS

- White rice – .75 cup
- Water – 1.5 cups
- Olive oil – 1.5 tablespoons
- Bay leaf, ground - .25 teaspoon
- Lime juice – 1 tablespoon
- Lemon juice – 1 tablespoon
- Lime zest - .25 teaspoon
- Cilantro, chopped - .25 cup

DIRECTIONS

1. Place the white rice and water in a medium-sized saucepan and bring it to a boil over medium heat. Simmer and cover the pot with a lid, allowing it to cook until all water has been absorbed about eighteen to twenty minutes.
2. Stir in the ground bay leaf, olive oil, lime juice, lemon juice, lime zest, and cilantro after cooking. You want to do this with a fork, preferably, as this will fluff the rice rather than causing it to compact. Serve while warm.

Nutritions: 363 Protein Grams: 5, Phosphorus Milligrams: 74, Potassium Milligrams: 86, Sodium Milligrams: 5, Fat Grams: 10, Total Carbohydrates Grams: 60, Net Carbohydrates Grams: 58

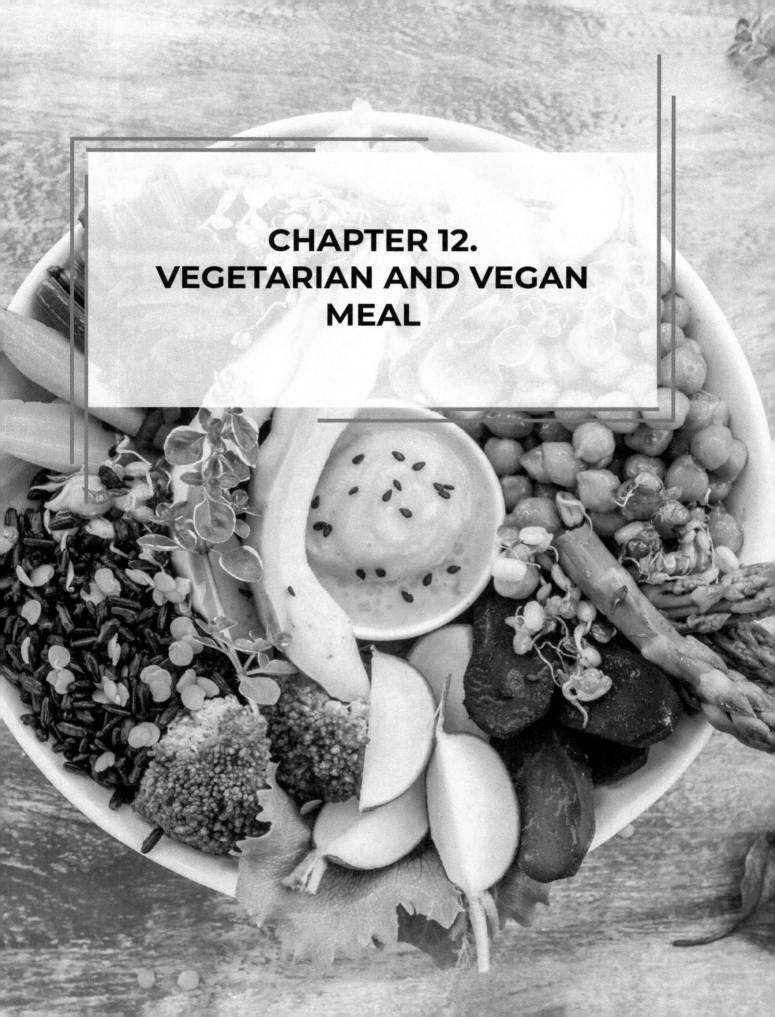

CHAPTER 12.
VEGETARIAN AND VEGAN MEAL

206. TOFU STIR FRY

PREPARATION: 15 MIN

COOKING: 20 MIN

SERVES: 4

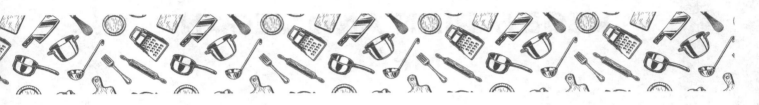

INGREDIENTS

- 1 teaspoon sugar
- 1 tablespoon lime juice
- 1 tablespoon low sodium soy sauce
- 2 tablespoons cornstarch
- 2 egg whites, beaten
- 1/2 cup unseasoned bread crumbs
- 1 tablespoon vegetable oil
- 16 ounces tofu, cubed
- 1 clove garlic, minced
- 1 tablespoon sesame oil
- 1 red bell pepper, sliced into strips
- 1 cup broccoli florets
- 1 teaspoon herb seasoning blend
- Dash black pepper
- Sesame seeds
- Steamed white rice

DIRECTIONS

1. Dissolve sugar in a mixture of lime juice and soy sauce. Set aside.
2. In the first bowl, put the cornstarch.
3. Add the egg whites in the second bowl.
4. Place the breadcrumbs in the third bowl.
5. Dip each tofu cubes in the first, second and third bowls.
6. Pour vegetable oil in a pan over medium heat.
7. Cook tofu cubes until golden.
8. Drain the tofu and set aside.
9. Remove oil from the pan and add sesame oil.
10. Add garlic, bell pepper and broccoli.
11. Cook until crisp tender.
12. Season with the seasoning blend and pepper.
13. Put the tofu back and toss to mix.
14. Pour soy sauce mixture on top and transfer to serving bowls.
15. Garnish with the sesame seeds and serve on top of white rice.

Nutritions: *Calories 401, Protein 19g, Carbohydrates 46g, Fat 16g, Cholesterol 0mg, Sodium 584mg, Potassium 317mg, Phosphorus 177mg, Calcium 253mg, Fiber 2.7g*

207. BROCCOLI PANCAKE

PREPARATION: 10 MIN

COOKING: 5 MIN

SERVES: 4

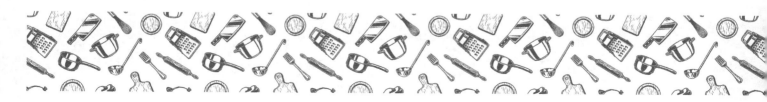

INGREDIENTS

- 3 cups broccoli florets, diced
- 2 eggs, beaten
- 2 tablespoons all-purpose flour
- 1/2 cup onion, chopped
- 2 tablespoons olive oil

DIRECTIONS

1. Boil broccoli in water for 5 minutes. Drain and set aside.
2. Mix egg and flour.
3. Add onion and broccoli to the mixture.
4. Cook the broccoli pancake until brown on both sides.

Nutritions: Calories 140, Protein 6g, Carbohydrates 7g, Fat 10g, Cholesterol 106mg, Sodium 58mg, Potassium 276mg, Phosphorus 101mg, Calcium 50mg, Fiber 2.1g

208. CARROT CASSEROLE

PREPARATION: 10 MIN

COOKING: 20 MIN

SERVES: 8

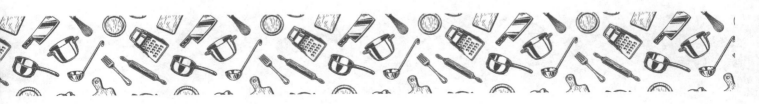

INGREDIENTS

- 1-pound carrots, sliced into rounds
- 12 low-sodium crackers
- 2 tablespoons butter
- 2 tablespoons onion, chopped
- 1/4 cup cheddar cheese, shredded

DIRECTIONS

1. Preheat your oven to 35o degrees f.
2. Boil the carrots in a pot of water until tender.
3. Drain the carrots and reserve ¼ cup liquid.
4. Mash carrots.
5. Add all the ingredients into the carrots except cheese.
6. Place the mashed carrots in a casserole dish.
7. Sprinkle cheese on top and bake in the oven for 15 minutes.

Nutritions: *Calories 97, Protein 2g, Carbohydrates 9g, Fat 7g, Cholesterol 13mg, Sodium 174mg, Potassium 153mg, Phosphorus 47mg, Calcium 66mg, Fiber 1.8g*

209. CAULIFLOWER RICE

PREPARATION: 10 MIN

COOKING: 10 MIN

SERVES: 4

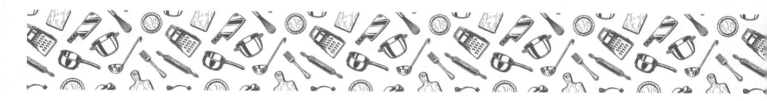

INGREDIENTS

- 1 head cauliflower, sliced into florets
- 1 tablespoon butter
- Black pepper to taste
- 1/4 teaspoon garlic powder
- 1/4 teaspoon herb seasoning blend

DIRECTIONS

1. Put cauliflower florets in a food processor.
2. Pulse until consistency is similar to grain.
3. In a pan of medium heat, melt the butter and add the spices.
4. Toss cauliflower rice and cook for 10 minutes.
5. Fluff using a fork before serving.

Nutritions: Calories 47, Protein 1g, Carbohydrates 4g, Fat 3g, Cholesterol 8mg, Sodium 43mg, Potassium 206mg, Phosphorus 31mg, Calcium 16mg, Fiber 1.4g

210. EGGPLANT FRIES

PREPARATION: 10 MIN

COOKING: 5 MIN

SERVES: 6

INGREDIENTS

- 2 eggs, beaten
- 1 cup almond milk
- 1 teaspoon hot sauce
- 3/4 cup cornstarch
- 3 teaspoons dry ranch seasoning mix
- 3/4 cup dry bread crumbs
- 1 eggplant, sliced into strips
- 1/2 cup oil

DIRECTIONS

1. In a bowl, mix eggs, milk and hot sauce.
2. In a dish, mix cornstarch, seasoning and breadcrumbs.
3. Dip first the eggplant strips in the egg mixture.
4. Coat each strip with the cornstarch mixture.
5. Pour oil in a pan over medium heat.
6. Once hot, add the fries and cook for 3 minutes or until golden.

Nutritions: *Calories 234, Protein 7g, Carbohydrates 25g, Fat 13g, Cholesterol 48mg, Sodium 212mg, Potassium 215mg, Phosphorus 86mg, Calcium 70mg, Fiber 2.1g*

211. SEASONED GREEN BEANS

PREPARATION: 10 MIN

COOKING: 10 MIN

SERVES: 4

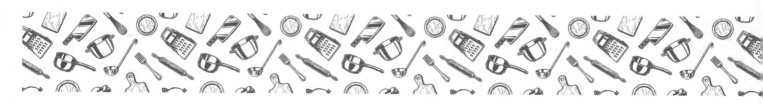

INGREDIENTS

- 10-ounce green beans
- 4 teaspoons butter
- 1/4 cup onion, chopped
- 1/2 cup red bell pepper, chopped
- 1 teaspoon dried dill weed
- 1 teaspoon dried parsley
- 1/4 teaspoon black pepper

DIRECTIONS

1. Boil the green beans in a pot of water. Drain.
2. In a pan of medium heat, melt the butter and cook onion and bell pepper.
3. Season with dill and parsley.
4. Put the green beans back to the skillet.
5. Sprinkle pepper on top before serving.

Nutritions: Calories 67, Protein 2g, Carbohydrates 8g, Fat 3g, Cholesterol 0mg, Sodium 55mg, Potassium 194mg, Phosphorus 32mg, Calcium 68mg, Fiber 4.0g

212. GRILLED SQUASH

PREPARATION: 10 MIN

COOKING: 6 MIN

SERVES: 8

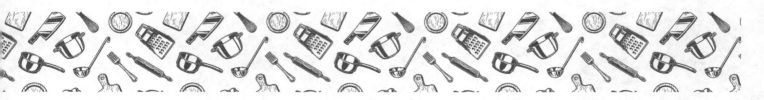

INGREDIENTS

- 4 zucchinis, rinsed, drained and sliced
- 4 crookneck squash, rinsed, drained and sliced
- Cooking spray
- 1/4 teaspoon garlic powder
- 1/4 teaspoon black pepper

DIRECTIONS

1. Arrange squash on a baking sheet.
2. Spray with oil.
3. Season with garlic powder and pepper.
4. Grill for 4 minutes per side or until tender but not too soft.

Nutritions: *Calories 17, Protein 1g, Carbohydrates 3g, Fat 0g, Cholesterol 0mg, Sodium 6mg, Potassium 262mg, Phosphorus 39mg, Calcium 16mg, Fiber 1.1g*

213. THAI TOFU BROTH

PREPARATION: 5 MIN

COOKING: 15 MIN

SERVES: 4

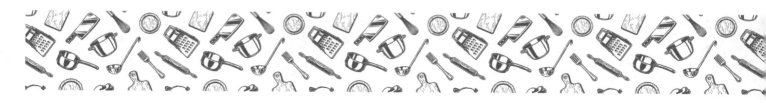

INGREDIENTS

- 1 cup rice noodles
- ½ sliced onion
- 6 ounce drained, pressed and cubed tofu
- ¼ cup sliced scallions
- ½ cup water
- ½ cup canned water chestnuts
- ½ cup rice milk
- 1 tablespoon lime juice
- 1 tablespoon coconut oil
- ½ finely sliced chili
- 1 cup snow peas

DIRECTIONS

1. Heat the oil in a wok on a high heat and then sauté the tofu until brown on each side.
2. Add the onion and sauté for 2-3 minutes.
3. Add the rice milk and water to the wok until bubbling.
4. Lower to medium heat and add the noodles, chili and water chestnuts.
5. Allow to simmer for 10-15 minutes and then add the sugar snap peas for 5 minutes.
6. Serve with a sprinkle of scallions.

Nutritions: Calories 304, Protein 9g, Carbs 38g, Fat 13g, Sodium (Na) 36mg, Potassium (K) 114mg, Phosphorus 101mg

214. DELICIOUS VEGETARIAN LASAGNA

PREPARATION: 10 MIN

COOKING: 1 H

SERVES: 4

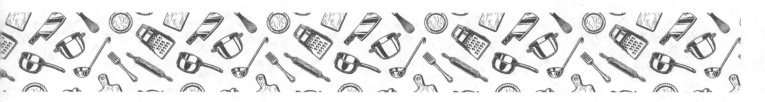

INGREDIENTS

- 1 teaspoon basil
- 1 tablespoon olive oil
- ½ sliced red pepper
- 3 lasagna sheets
- ½ diced red onion
- ¼ teaspoon black pepper
- 1 cup rice milk
- 1 minced garlic clove
- 1 cup sliced eggplant
- ½ sliced zucchini
- ½ pack soft tofu
- 1 teaspoon oregano

DIRECTIONS

1. Preheat oven to 325°f/gas mark 3.
2. Slice zucchini, eggplant and pepper into vertical strips.
3. Add the rice milk and tofu to a food processor and blitz until smooth. Set aside.
4. Heat the oil in a skillet over medium heat and add the onions and garlic for 3-4 minutes or until soft.
5. Sprinkle in the herbs and pepper and allow to stir through for 5-6 minutes until hot.
6. Into a lasagna or suitable oven dish, layer 1 lasagna sheet, then 1/3 the eggplant, followed by 1/3 zucchini, then 1/3 pepper before pouring over 1/3 of tofu white sauce.
7. Repeat for the next 2 layers, finishing with the white sauce.
8. Add to the oven for 40-50 minutes or until veg is soft and can easily be sliced into servings.

Nutritions: *Calories 235, Protein 5g, Carbs 10g, Fat 9g, Sodium (Na) 35mg, Potassium (K) 129mg, Phosphorus 66mg*

215. CHILI TOFU NOODLES

PREPARATION: 5 MIN

COOKING: 15 MIN

SERVES: 4

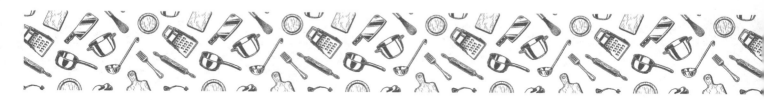

INGREDIENTS

- ½ diced red chili
- 2 cups rice noodles
- ½ juiced lime
- 6 ounce pressed and cubed silken firm tofu
- 1 teaspoon grated fresh ginger
- 1 tablespoon coconut oil
- 1 cup green beans
- 1 minced garlic clove

DIRECTIONS

1. Steam the green beans for 10-12 minutes or according to package directions and drain.
2. Cook the noodles in a pot of boiling water for 10-15 minutes or according to package directions.
3. Meanwhile, heat a wok or skillet on a high heat and add coconut oil.
4. Now add the tofu, chili flakes, garlic and ginger and sauté for 5-10 minutes.
5. After doing that, drain in the noodles along with the green beans and lime juice then add it to the wok.
6. Toss to coat.
7. Serve hot!

Nutritions: Calories 246, Protein 10g, Carbs 28g, Fat 12g, Sodium (Na) 25mg, Potassium (K) 126mg, Phosphorus 79mg

216. CURRIED CAULIFLOWER

PREPARATION: 5 MIN

COOKING: 20 MIN

SERVES: 4

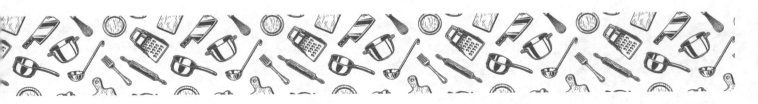

INGREDIENTS

- 1 teaspoon turmeric
- 1 diced onion
- 1 tablespoon chopped fresh cilantro
- 1 teaspoon cumin
- ½ diced chili
- ½ cup water
- 1 minced garlic clove
- 1 tablespoon coconut oil
- 1 teaspoon garam masala
- 2 cups cauliflower florets

DIRECTIONS

1. Add the oil to a skillet on medium heat.
2. Sauté the onion and garlic for 5 minutes until soft.
3. Add in the cumin, turmeric and garam masala and stir to release the aromas.
4. Now add the chili to the pan along with the cauliflower.
5. Stir to coat.
6. Pour in the water and reduce the heat to a simmer for 15 minutes.
7. Garnish with cilantro to serve.

Nutritions: *Calories 108, Protein 2g, Carbs 11g, Fat 7g, Sodium (Na) 35mg, Potassium (K) 328mg, Phosphorus 39mg*

217. SIMPLE BROCCOLI STIR-FRY

 PREPARATION: 40 MIN

 COOKING: 15 MIN

 SERVES: 4

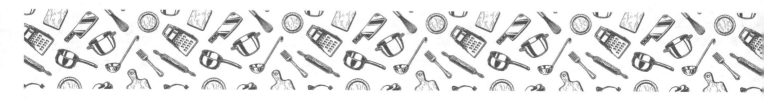

INGREDIENTS

- 1 tablespoon of olive oil
- 1 minced garlic clove
- 2 cups of broccoli florets
- 2 tablespoons of water

DIRECTIONS

1. Heat oil on medium heat.
2. Add garlic and then sauté for about 1 minute.
3. Add the broccoli and stir fry for about 2 minutes.
4. Stir in water and stir fry for about 4-5 minutes.
5. Serve warm.

Nutritions: Calories: 47, Fat: 3.6g, Carbs: 3.3g, Protein: 1.3g, Fiber: 1.2g, Potassium: 147mg, Sodium: 15mg

218. BRAISED CABBAGE

PREPARATION: 30 MIN

COOKING: 15 MIN

SERVES: 4

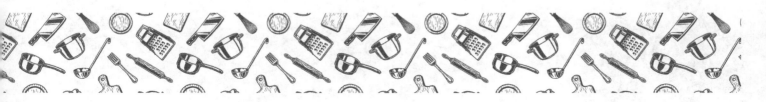

INGREDIENTS

- 1½ teaspoon of olive oil
- 2 minced garlic cloves
- 1 thinly sliced onion
- 3 cups of chopped green cabbage
- 1 cup of low-sodium vegetable broth
- Freshly ground black pepper, to taste

DIRECTIONS

1. In a large skillet, heat oil on medium-high heat.
2. Add garlic and then sauté for about 1 minute.
3. Add onion and sauté for about 4-5 minutes.
4. Add cabbage and sauté for about 3-4 minutes.
5. Stir in broth and black pepper and immediately, reduce the heat to low.
6. Cook, covered for about 20 minutes.
7. Serve warm.

Nutritions: *Calories: 45, Fat: 1.8g, Carbs: 6.6g, Protein: 1.1g, Fiber: 1.9g, Potassium: 136mg, Sodium: 46mg*

219. SALAD WITH STRAWBERRIES AND GOAT CHEESE

PREPARATION: 15 MIN

COOKING: 0 MIN

SERVES: 2

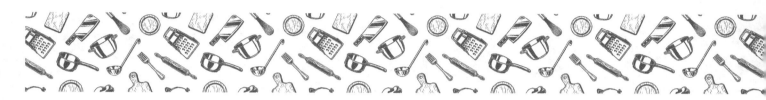

INGREDIENTS

- Baby lettuce, to taste
- 1-pint strawberries
- Balsamic vinegar
- Extra virgin olive oil
- 1/4 teaspoon black pepper
- 8-ounce soft goat cheese

DIRECTIONS

1. Prepare the lettuce by washing and drying it, then cut the strawberries.
2. Cut the soft goat cheese into 8 pieces.
3. Put together the balsamic vinegar and the extra virgin olive oil in a large cup with a whisk.
4. Mix the strawberries pressing them and putting them in a bowl, add the dressing and mix, then divide the lettuce into four dishes and cut the other strawberries, arranging them on the salad.
5. Put cheese slices on top and add pepper. Serve and enjoy!

Nutritions: Calories: 300, Protein: 13g, Sodium: 285mg, Potassium: 400mg, Phosphorus: 193 Mg

220. ROASTED VEGGIES MEDITERRANEAN STYLE

PREPARATION: 5 MIN

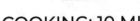

COOKING: 10 MIN

SERVES: 2

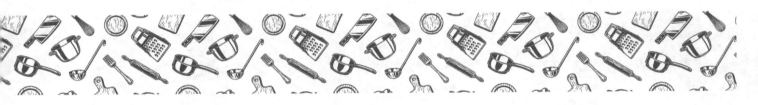

INGREDIENTS

- ½ teaspoon freshly grated lemon zest
- 1 cup grape tomatoes
- 1 tablespoon extra-virgin olive oil
- 1 tablespoon lemon juice
- 1 teaspoon dried oregano
- 10 pitted black olives, sliced
- 12-ounce broccoli crowns, trimmed and cut into bite-sized pieces
- 2 cloves garlic, minced
- 2 teaspoons capers, rinsed

DIRECTIONS

1. Preheat oven to 350of and grease a baking sheet with cooking spray.
2. In a large bowl toss together until thoroughly coated salt, garlic, oil, tomatoes and broccoli. Spread broccoli on prepped baking sheet and bake for 8 to 10 minutes.
3. In another large bowl mix capers, oregano, olives, lemon juice, and lemon zest. Mix in roasted vegetables and serve while still warm.

Nutritions: *Calories: 110; Carbs: 16g; Protein: 6g; Fats: 4g; Phosphorus: 138mg; Potassium: 745mg; Sodium: 214mg*

221. FRUITY GARDEN LETTUCE SALAD

PREPARATION: 10 MIN

COOKING: 0 MIN

SERVES: 4

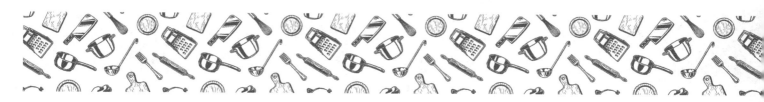

INGREDIENTS

- ¼ cup apple cider vinegar
- ¼ cup chopped almonds
- ½ avocado, thinly sliced
- ½ cup extra virgin olive oil
- ½ lemon, juiced
- 1 teaspoon ground black pepper
- 2 granny smith apples, thinly sliced
- 2 teaspoons grainy mustard
- 6 cups thinly sliced lettuce

DIRECTIONS

1. In a large salad bowl, toss lemon juice and apples. Mix in almonds, avocado, and lettuce.
2. Mix salt, pepper, mustard, vinegar and olive oil until salt is thoroughly dissolved.
3. Pour in the dressing all over lettuce mixture and toss well to combine. Serve and enjoy.

Nutritions: Calories: 123; Carbs: 16.5g; Protein: 2g; Fats: 6g; Phosphorus: 56mg; Potassium: 450mg; Sodium: 35mg

222. BAKED DILLY PICKEREL

PREPARATION: 5 MIN

COOKING: 15 MIN

SERVES: 3

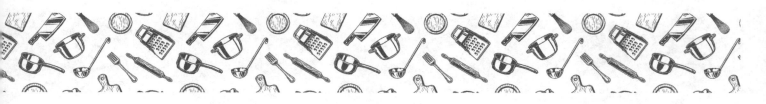

INGREDIENTS

- 4 fillets of pickerel, about 4 ounces
- For the dilly sauce
- ½ package of whipped cream cheese
- 4 minced garlic cloves
- ½ diced small onion
- 3 tablespoons of fresh or dried dill
- ½ teaspoon of ground pepper

DIRECTIONS

1. Preheat your oven to a temperature of 345°f.
2. Mix the ingredients of the dilly sauce very well to make a paste.
3. Line a baking pan with a tin foil; then set the fish and spread the dilly sauce on its top
4. Cover the fish with an aluminum foil tin and bake it for about 15 minutes in the oven
5. Serve and enjoy your dinner!

Nutritions: *Calories: 295.6, Fats: 18.7g, Carbs: 11g, Fiber: 2.2g, Potassium: 140mg, Sodium: 6.8mg, Phosphorous: 58g, Protein 20.7g*

223. RICE SALAD

PREPARATION: 10 MIN

COOKING: 20 MIN

SERVES: 2

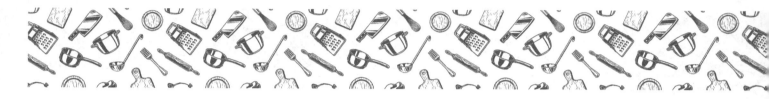

INGREDIENTS

- 1 cup of olive oil
- ½ cup of balsamic vinegar
- 1 teaspoon of lemon juice
- ¾ teaspoons of black pepper
- 3 minced garlic cloves
- ½ teaspoon of dried basil
- ½ teaspoon of dried oregano
- ½ cup of fresh parsley
- 2 cups of bell peppers
- ½ cup of chopped red onion
- 1 cup of frozen artichoke hearts
- 1/3 cup of fresh dill weed
- 6 cups of cooked white rice
- 1 pound of cooked shrimp
- ½ cup of dried cranberries
- 8 ounces of canned pineapple chunks
- 1 cup of frozen green peas

DIRECTIONS

1. To make the dressing, whisk all together the oil with the vinegar, the salt, the pepper, the minced garlic, the basil, the oregano and about ¼ cup of chopped parsley; then set the mixture aside.
2. Chop the red bell peppers and the onion; then mince the dill weed
3. Cook your ingredients and quarter the artichoke hearts.
4. In a large bowl combine the rice with the shrimp, the bell peppers, the onion, the artichoke hearts, and ½ cup of minced parsley, the dill, the cranberries, the pineapple and the green peas.
5. Stir the dressing and let it chill for about 2 hours to marinate.
6. Serve and enjoy your dinner over a bed of lettuce!

Nutritions: Calories: 165.4, Fats: 11g, Carbs: 8g, Fiber: 0.89g, Potassium: 181mg, Sodium:99mg, Phosphorous: 75g, Protein 8g

224. BAKED EGGPLANT TRAY

PREPARATION: 10 MIN

COOKING: 20 MIN

SERVES: 2

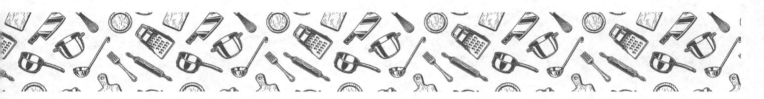

INGREDIENTS

- 3 cups of eggplant
- 3 large omega-3 eggs
- ½ cup of liquid non-dairy creamer
- 1 teaspoon of vinegar
- 1 teaspoon of lemon juice
- ½ teaspoon of pepper
- ¼ teaspoon of sage
- ½ cup of white breadcrumbs
- 1 tablespoon of margarine

DIRECTIONS

1. Preheat the oven to a temperature of about 350° f
2. Peel the eggplant and cut it into pieces
3. Place the eggplant pieces in a large pan; then cover it with water and let boil until it becomes tender
4. Drain the eggplants and mash it very well
5. Combine the beaten eggs with the non-dairy creamer, the vinegar, the lemon juice, the pepper and the sage with the mashed eggplant; then place it into a greased baking tray
6. Mix the melted margarine with the breadcrumbs.
7. Top you tray with the breadcrumbs and bake it for about 20 minutes
8. Set the tray aside to cool for about 5 minutes
9. Serve and enjoy your dinner!

Nutritions: *Calories: 126, Fats: 8g, Carbs: 4.7g, Fiber: 1.6g, Potassium: 224mg, Sodium: 143mg, Phosphorous: 115g, Protein 7.3g*

225. RAW VEGETABLES. CHOPPED SALAD

PREPARATION: 15 MIN **COOKING: 0 MIN** **SERVES: 4**

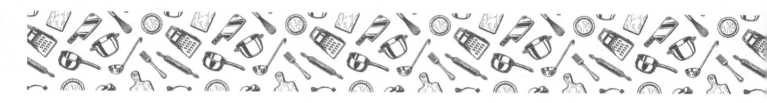

INGREDIENTS

- Chopped raw veggie salad
- 1 orange pepper (minced) (about 1 cup)
- 1 yellow pepper (small cut) (about 1 cup)
- 5-8 radishes (halve and cut into thin slices) (about 3/4 cup)
- Small head of broccoli (minced) (about 2 cups)
- 1 seedless cucumber (small cut) (about 2 cups)
- 1 cup of halved red seedless grapes
- 2-3 tablespoons chopped fresh dill
- 1/4 cup chopped fresh parsley
- 1/4 cup of raw peeled sunflower seeds
- 1/8 cup raw hemp hearts (peeled hemp seeds)
- Oil-free dressing
- Garlic clove (chopped)
- Tablespoons of red wine vinegar
- 1 tablespoon of apple cider vinegar
- Juice of 1 lemon
- 1 tablespoon dijonsenf
- 1 tablespoon pure maple syrup
- 1/2 teaspoon salt (or to taste)
- 1/8 teaspoon pepper (or to taste)

DIRECTIONS

1. Whisk the ingredients - chopped raw veggie salad, 1 orange pepper, yellow pepper, radishes, small head of broccoli, seedless cucumber, halved red seedless grapes, chopped fresh dill, chopped fresh parsley, raw peeled sunflower seeds, raw hemp hearts, garlic clove, red wine vinegar, apple cider vinegar, lemon, dijonsenf, pure maple syrup, salt, pepper. For dressing in a small bowl and set aside.
2. Mix all the salad ingredients in a large bowl.
3. Pour the dressing over and wrap well.
4. Cover and then refrigerate it for an hour or two and toss the salad once or twice during this time to coat evenly. Enjoy!

Nutritions: Calories: 111, Total Fat: 2g, Saturated Fat: 1g, Cholesterol: 10mg, Sodium: 58mg, Carbohydrates: 19g, Sugar: 18g, Calcium: 15%

226. MEDITERRANEAN VEGGIE PITA SANDWICH

PREPARATION: 4 H 30 MIN

COOKING: 30 MIN

SERVES: 2

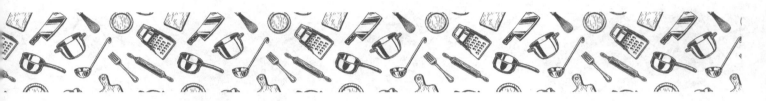

INGREDIENTS

- 1/4 cup chopped carrots
- A handful of baby spinach
- 1/4 cup chickpeas
- 1 teaspoon of crumbled feta cheese
- 2 teaspoons of fine chopped sun-dried tomatoes
- 2 teaspoons of chopped kalamata olives
- Season with salt and pepper

DIRECTIONS

1. The chopped carrots, baby spinach, chickpeas, crumbled feta cheese, chopped sun-dried tomatoes, chopped kalamata olives, salt and pepper. Spread the bath in every pita pant. Sort the rest of the ingredients between the boxes. Eat immediately or pack in a container for lunch. Cool the device if you prepare it for more than 4 hours before eating.

Nutritions: *Calories 287.6, Sodium 716.0mg, Potassium 263.6mg, Total Carbohydrate 45.7g, Dietary Fiber 6.8g*

227. CLASSIC ASPARAGUS

PREPARATION: 20 MIN

COOKING: 20 MIN

SERVES: 4

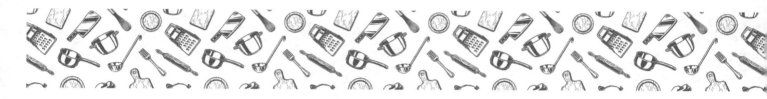

INGREDIENTS

- 2 kg of white asparagus
- 12 pieces medium potatoes
- 4 eggs
- 1 first-class salt
- 1 premium sugar
- 1 tablespoon butter
- For the sauce:
- 200 g butter
- 2 egg yolks
- 4 tablespoons white wine
- 1 tablespoon lemon juice
- 1 first-class salt
- 1 premium white pepper

DIRECTIONS

1. Cook the peeled asparagus in plenty of hot water (seasoned with salt, sugar, and butter) for 15 - 20 minutes.
2. Peel the potatoes and cook as usual or cool with the air freezer. The eggs are cooked hard.
3. For the sauce: dissolve the butter in a hot freezer and allow cooling slightly.
4. Grease the egg yolks with lemon juice and white wine in a warm water bath until the mass is thick.
5. Then the cooled and melted butter is slowed down slowly. Now the sauce is seasoned with salt and pepper.
6. Tips on the recipe
7. Distribute the asparagus in 4 portions and arrange with potatoes and the halved eggs on 4 plates.

Nutritions: Calories 20%, Daily Value Total Fat 0.1g 0%, Saturated Fat 0g 0%, Total Carbohydrate 3.9g, 1% Dietary Fiber 2.1g 8%, Sugar 1.9g, Protein 2.2g 4%

228. VEGETARIAN PASTICCIO

PREPARATION: 10 MIN

COOKING: 30 MIN

SERVES: 4

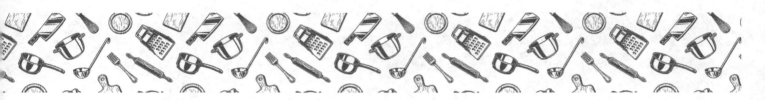

INGREDIENTS

- 7 eggs
- 7 slices of sourdough bread
- 1-ounce shredded sharp cheddar cheese
- 1 piece of onion
- 1 cup of raw mushrooms
- 1 cup red bell peppers
- 15 fresh spinach leaves
- ½ teaspoon black pepper
- ¼ glass vinegar§
- 3 portions of half and half cream
- Worcestershire sauce (1 teaspoon)
- Hot sauce (1 teaspoon)
- Unsalted margarine (1 teaspoon)

DIRECTIONS

1. Cut onion, pepper and mushrooms into small dices.
2. Chop bread into small dices and place on a baking sheet. Bake in the oven at 225°f (or 100°c) for 15 minutes, turning the cubes every 15 minutes and then still cook them for other 15 minutes.
3. Put onion, pepper and mushrooms mix in a skillet pre-greased with olive oil.
4. Grease a dish and put in it both bread dices and the vegetable mixture, then put the spinach leaves on top. Arrange for a second layer of the same mixture.
5. Put together the half and half cream with eggs, vinegar, worcestershire sauce, hot sauce and black pepper. Pour this mix over the bread. Put the covered dish in the fridge for one hour. When out of the fridge, put the dish aside for at least 20 minutes.
6. Preheat oven at 330 °f. Bake for 50 minutes without the covering and when you take it out of the oven, sprinkle the cheddar cheese over the top. Cook for 10 minutes and cut into 10 slices and serve it hot.

Nutritions: *210 calories 10g, protein 15g, carbohydrates 10g, fat 165mg, cholesterol 215mg, sodium 345mg, potassium 205mg, phosphorus 150mg, calcium 2.0 fiber*

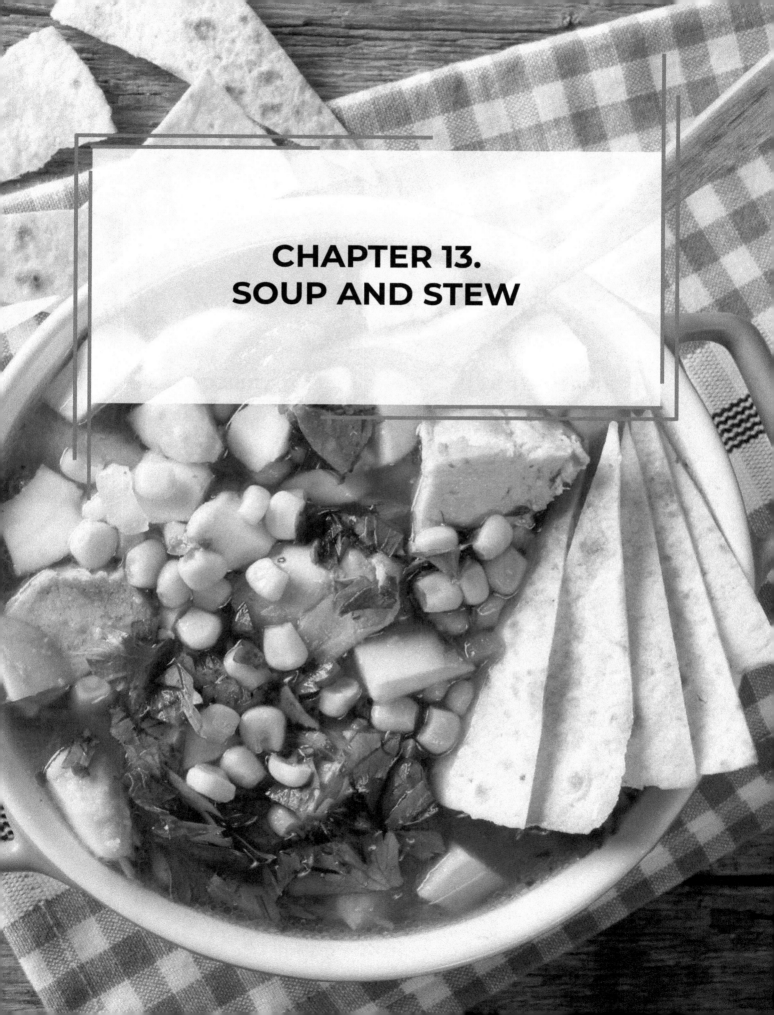

CHAPTER 13.
SOUP AND STEW

229. CHICKEN WILD RICE SOUP

PREPARATION: 10 MIN

COOKING: 15 MIN

SERVES: 6

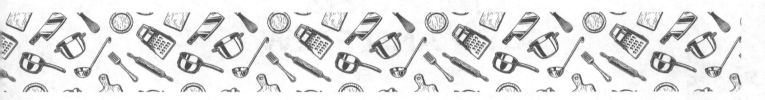

INGREDIENTS

- 2/3 cup wild rice, uncooked
- 1 tablespoon onion, chopped finely
- 1 tablespoon fresh parsley, chopped
- 1 cup carrots, chopped
- 8-ounce chicken breast, cooked
- 2 tablespoon butter
- 1/4 cup all-purpose white flour
- 5 cups low-sodium chicken broth
- 1 tablespoon slivered almonds

DIRECTIONS

1. Start by adding rice and 2 cups broth along with ½ cup water to a cooking pot.
2. Cook the chicken until the rice is al dente and set it aside.
3. Add butter to a saucepan and melt it.
4. Stir in onion and sauté until soft then add the flour and the remaining broth.
5. Stir it and then cook for it 1 minute then add the chicken, cooked rice, and carrots.
6. Cook for 5 minutes on simmer.
7. Garnish with almonds.
8. Serve fresh.

Nutritions: *Calories 287. Protein 21 g. Carbohydrates 35 g. Fat 7 g. Cholesterol 42 mg. Sodium 182 mg. Potassium 384 mg. Phosphorus 217 mg. Calcium 45 mg. Fiber 1.6 g.*

230. CHICKEN NOODLE SOUP

PREPARATION: 10 MIN

COOKING: 25 MIN

SERVES: 2

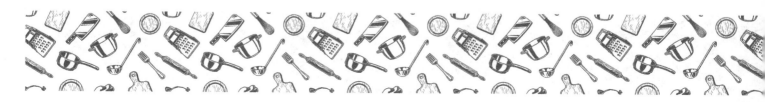

INGREDIENTS

- 1 1/2 cups low-sodium vegetable broth
- 1 cup of water
- 1/4 teaspoon poultry seasoning
- 1/4 teaspoon black pepper
- 1 cup chicken strips
- 1/4 cup carrot
- 2-ounce egg noodles, uncooked

DIRECTIONS

1. Gather all the ingredients into a slow cooker and toss it
2. Cook soup on high heat for 25 minutes.
3. Serve warm.

Nutritions: Calories 103. Protein 8 g. Carbohydrates 11 g. Fat 3 g. Cholesterol 4 mg. Sodium 355 mg. Potassium 264 mg. Phosphorus 128 mg. Calcium 46 mg. Fiber 4.0 g.

231. CUCUMBER SOUP

PREPARATION: 10 MIN **COOKING: 0 MIN** **SERVES: 4**

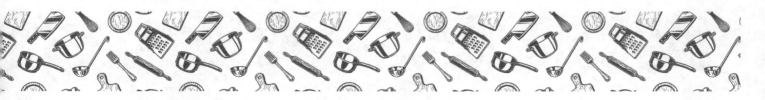

INGREDIENTS

- 2 medium cucumbers, peeled and diced
- 1/3 cup sweet white onion, diced
- 1 green onion, diced
- 1/4 cup fresh mint
- 2 tablespoon fresh dill
- 2 tablespoon lemon juice
- 2/3 cup water
- 1/2 cup half and half cream
- 1/3 cup sour cream
- 1/2 teaspoon pepper
- Fresh dill sprigs for garnish

DIRECTIONS

1. Gather all of the ingredients into a food processor and toss.
2. Puree the mixture and refrigerate for 2 hours.
3. Garnish with dill sprigs.
4. Enjoy fresh.

Nutritions: *Calories 77. Protein 2 g. Carbohydrates 6 g. Fat 5 g. Cholesterol 12 mg. Sodium 128 mg. Potassium 258 mg. Phosphorus 64 mg. Calcium 60 mg. Fiber 1.0 g.*

232. SQUASH AND TURMERIC SOUP

PREPARATION: 10 MIN

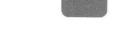

COOKING: 30 MIN

SERVES: 4

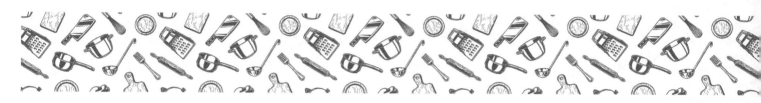

INGREDIENTS

- 4 cups low-sodium vegetable broth
- 2 medium zucchini squash, peeled and diced
- 2 medium yellow crookneck squash, peeled and diced
- 1 small onion, diced
- 1/2 cup frozen green peas
- 2 tablespoon olive oil
- 1/2 cup plain nonfat Greek yogurt
- 2 teaspoon turmeric

DIRECTIONS

1. Warm the broth in a saucepan on medium heat.
2. Toss in onion, squash, and zucchini.
3. Let it simmer for approximately 25 minutes then add oil and green peas.
4. Cook for another 5 minutes then allow it to cool.
5. Puree the soup using a handheld blender then add Greek yogurt and turmeric.
6. Refrigerate it overnight and serve fresh.

Nutritions: Calories 100. Protein 4 g. Carbohydrates 10 g. Fat 5 g. Cholesterol 1 mg. Sodium 279 mg. Potassium 504 mg. Phosphorus 138 mg. Calcium 60 mg. Fiber 2.8 g.

233. LEEK, POTATO AND CARROT SOUP

PREPARATION: 15 MIN

COOKING: 25 MIN

SERVES: 4

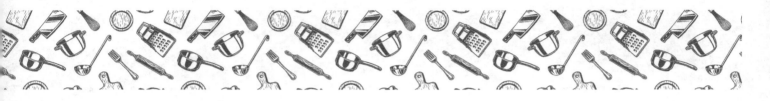

INGREDIENTS

- 1 - leek
- ¾ - cup diced and boiled potatoes
- ¾ - cup diced and boiled carrots
- 1 - garlic clove
- 1 - tablespoon oil
- crushed pepper to taste
- 3 - cups low sodium chicken stock
- chopped parsley for garnish
- 1 - bay leaf
- ¼ - teaspoon ground cumin

DIRECTIONS

1. Trim off and take away a portion of the course inexperienced portions of the leek, at that factor reduce daintily and flush altogether in virus water.
2. Channel properly. Warmth the oil in an extensively based pot.
3. Include the leek and garlic, and sear over low warmth for two-3 minutes, till sensitive.
4. Include the inventory, inlet leaf, cumin, and pepper. Heat the mixture, mix constantly.
5. Include the bubbled potatoes and carrots and stew for 10-15minutes
6. Modify the flavoring, eliminate the inlet leaf and serve sprinkled generously with slashed parsley.
7. To make a pureed soup, manner the soup in a blender or nourishment processor till smooth
8. Come again to the pan. Include ½ field milk.
9. Bring to bubble and stew for 2-3minutes

Nutritions: *Calories 315g, Fat 8g, Carbs 15g, Sugars 1.2g, Protein 26g*

234. ROASTED RED PEPPER SOUP

PREPARATION: 30 MIN

COOKING: 35 MIN

SERVES: 4

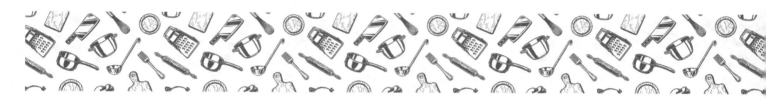

INGREDIENTS

- 4 - cups low-sodium chicken broth
- 3 - red peppers
- 2 - medium onions
- 3 - tablespoon lemon juice
- 1 - tablespoon finely minced lemon zest
- A pinch cayenne peppers
- ¼ - teaspoon cinnamon
- ½ - cup finely minced fresh cilantro

DIRECTIONS

1. In a medium stockpot, consolidate each one of the fixings except for the cilantro and warmth to the point of boiling over excessive warm temperature.
2. Diminish the warmth and stew, ordinarily secured, for around 30 minutes, till thickened.
3. Cool marginally. Utilizing a hand blender or nourishment processor, puree the soup.
4. Include the cilantro and tenderly heat.

Nutritions: Calories 265g, Fat 8g, Carbs 5g, Sugars 0.1g, Protein 29g

235. YUCATAN SOUP

PREPARATION: 10 MIN

COOKING: 20 MIN

SERVES: 4

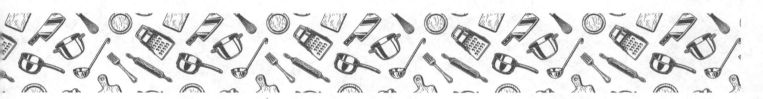

INGREDIENTS

- ½ cup onion, chopped
- 8 cloves garlic, chopped
- 2 Serrano chili peppers, chopped
- 1 medium tomato, chopped
- 1 ½ cups chicken breast, cooked, shredded
- 2 six-inch corn tortillas, sliced
- Nonstick cooking spray
- 1 tablespoon olive oil
- 4 cups chicken broth
- 1 bay leaf
- ¼ cup lime juice
- ¼ cup cilantro, chopped
- 1 teaspoon black pepper

DIRECTIONS

1. Spread the corn tortillas in a baking sheet and bake them for 3 minutes at 400°F.
2. Place a suitably-sized saucepan over medium heat and add oil to heat.
3. Toss in chili peppers, garlic, and onion, then sauté until soft.
4. Stir in broth, tomatoes, bay leaf, and chicken.
5. Let this chicken soup cook for 10 minutes on a simmer.
6. Stir in cilantro, lime juice, and black pepper.
7. Garnish with baked corn tortillas.
8. Serve.

Nutritions: *Calories: 215, Protein: 21 g, Carbohydrates: 32 g, Fat: 10 g, Cholesterol: 32 mg, Sodium: 246 mg, Potassium: 355 mg, Phosphorus: 176 mg, Calcium: 47 mg, Fiber: 1.6 g*

236. ZESTY TACO SOUP

PREPARATION: 10 MIN

COOKING: 7 H

SERVES: 2

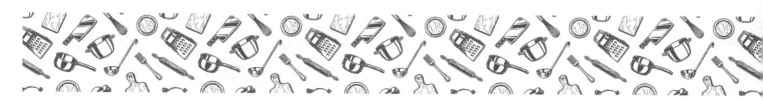

INGREDIENTS

- 1 ½ pounds boneless skinless chicken breast
- 15 ½ ounces canned dark red kidney beans
- 15 ½ ounces canned white corn
- 1 cup canned tomatoes, diced
- ½ cup onion
- 15 ½ ounces canned yellow hominy
- ½ cup green bell peppers
- 1 garlic clove
- 1 medium jalapeno
- 1 tablespoon package McCormick
- 2 cups chicken broth

DIRECTIONS

1. Add drained beans, hominy, corn, onion, garlic, jalapeno pepper, chicken, and green peppers to a Crockpot.
2. Cover the beans-corn mixture and cook for 1 hour on High temperature.
3. Reduce the heat to LOW and continue cooking for 6 hours.
4. Shred the slow-cooked chicken and return to the taco soup.
5. Serve warm.

Nutritions: Calories: 191, Protein: 21 g, Carbohydrates: 20 g, Fat: 3 g, Cholesterol: 42 mg, Sodium: 421 mg, Potassium: 444 mg, Phosphorus: 210 mg, Calcium: 28 mg, Fiber: 4.3 g

237. SOUTHWESTERN POSOLE

PREPARATION: 10 MIN

COOKING: 53 MIN

SERVES: 4

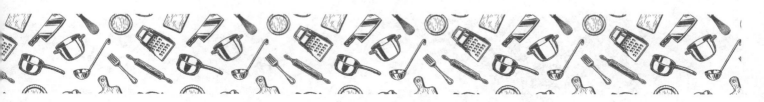

INGREDIENTS

- 1 tablespoon olive oil
- 1-pound pork loin, diced
- ½ cup onion, chopped
- 1 garlic clove, chopped
- 28 ounces canned white hominy
- 4 ounces canned diced green chilis
- 4 cups chicken broth
- ¼ teaspoon black pepper

DIRECTIONS

1. Place a suitably-sized cooking pot over medium heat and add oil to heat.
2. Toss in pork pieces and sauté for 4 minutes.
3. Stir in garlic and onion, then stir for 4 minutes, or until onion is soft.
4. Add the remaining ingredients, then cover the pork soup.
5. Cook this for 45 minutes, or until the pork is tender.
6. Serve warm.

Nutritions: *Calories: 286, Protein: 25 g, Carbohydrates: 15 g, Fat: 13 g, Cholesterol: 63 mg, Sodium: 399 mg, Potassium: 346 mg, Phosphorus: 182 mg, Calcium: 31 mg, Fiber: 3.4 g*

238. SPRING VEGETABLE SOUP

PREPARATION: 10 MIN

COOKING: 45 MIN

SERVES: 4

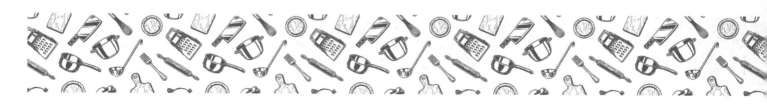

INGREDIENTS

- 1 cup fresh green beans, chopped
- ¾ cup celery, chopped
- ½ cup onion, chopped
- ½ cup carrots, chopped
- ½ cup mushrooms, chopped
- ½ cup frozen corn
- 1 medium Roma tomato, chopped
- 2 tablespoons olive oil
- ½ cup frozen corn
- 4 cups vegetable broth
- 1 teaspoon dried oregano leaves
- 1 teaspoon garlic powder

DIRECTIONS

1. Place a suitably-sized cooking pot over medium heat and add olive oil to heat.
2. Toss in onion and celery, then sauté until soft.
3. Stir in the corn and rest of the ingredients and cook the soup to boil.
4. Now reduce its heat to a simmer and cook for 45 minutes.
5. Serve warm.

Nutritions: Calories: 115, Protein: 3 g, Carbohydrates: 13 g, Fat: 6 g, Cholesterol: 0 mg, Sodium: 262 mg, Potassium: 400 mg, Phosphorus: 108 mg, Calcium: 48 mg, Fiber: 3.4 g

239. SEAFOOD CORN CHOWDER

PREPARATION: 10 MIN

COOKING: 12 MIN

SERVES: 4

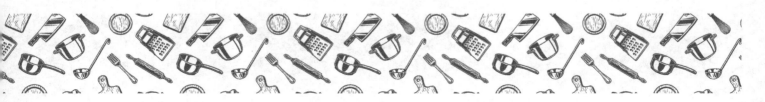

INGREDIENTS

- 1 tablespoon butter
- 1 cup onion, chopped
- 1/3 cup celery, chopped
- ½ cup green bell pepper, chopped
- ½ cup red bell pepper, chopped
- 1 tablespoon white flour
- 14 ounces chicken broth
- 2 cups cream
- 6 ounces evaporated milk
- 10 ounces surimi imitation crab chunks
- 2 cups frozen corn kernels
- ½ teaspoon black pepper
- ½ teaspoon paprika

DIRECTIONS

1. Place a suitably-sized saucepan over medium heat and add butter to melt.
2. Toss in onion, green and red peppers, and celery, then sauté for 5 minutes.
3. Stir in flour and whisk well for 2 minutes.
4. Pour in chicken broth and stir until it boils.
5. Add evaporated milk, corn, surimi crab, paprika, black pepper, and creamer.
6. Cook for 5 minutes then serve warm.

Nutritions: *Calories: 175, Protein: 8 g, Carbohydrates: 24 g, Fat: 7 g, Cholesterol: 13 mg, Sodium: 160 mg, Potassium: 285 mg, Phosphorus: 181 mg, Calcium: 68 mg, Fiber: 1.5 g*

240. BEEF SAGE SOUP

PREPARATION: 10 MIN

COOKING: 20 MIN

SERVES: 4

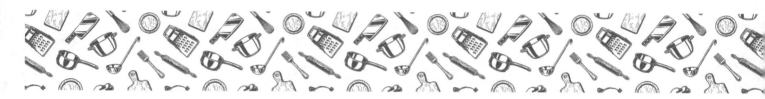

INGREDIENTS

- ½ pound ground beef
- ½ teaspoon ground sage
- ½ teaspoon black pepper
- ½ teaspoon dried basil
- ½ teaspoon garlic powder
- 4 slices bread, cubed
- 2 tablespoons olive oil
- 1 tablespoon herb seasoning blend
- 2 garlic cloves, minced
- 3 cups chicken broth
- 1 ½ cups water
- 4 tablespoons fresh parsley
- 2 tablespoons parmesan cheese, grated

DIRECTIONS

1. Preheat your oven to 375°F.
2. Mix beef with sage, basil, black pepper, and garlic powder in a bowl, then set it aside.
3. Toss the bread cubes with olive oil in a baking sheet and bake them for 8 minutes.
4. Meanwhile, sauté the beef mixture in a greased cooking pot until it is browned.
5. Stir in garlic and sauté for 2 minutes, then add parsley, water, and broth.
6. Cover the beef soup and cook for 10 minutes on a simmer.
7. Garnish the soup with parmesan cheese and baked bread.
8. Serve warm.

Nutritions: Calories: 336, Protein: 26 g, Carbohydrates: 16 g, Fat: 19 g, Cholesterol: 250 mg, Sodium: 374 mg, Potassium: 392 mg, Phosphorus: 268 mg, Calcium: 118 mg, Fiber: 0.9 g

241. CABBAGE BORSCHT

PREPARATION: 10 MIN

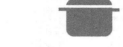

COOKING: 1 H 30 MIN

SERVES: 6

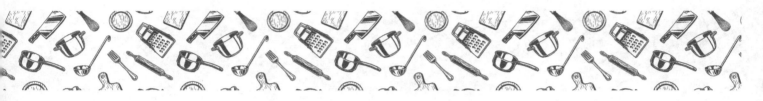

INGREDIENTS

- 2 pounds beef steaks
- 6 cups cold water
- 2 tablespoons olive oil
- ½ cup tomato sauce
- 1 medium cabbage, chopped
- 1 cup onion, diced
- 1 cup carrots, diced
- 1 cup turnips, peeled and diced
- 1 teaspoon pepper
- 6 tablespoons lemon juice
- 4 tablespoons sugar

DIRECTIONS

1. Start by placing steak in a large cooking pot and pour enough water to cover it.
2. Cover the beef pot and cook it on a simmer until it is tender, then shred it using a fork.
3. Add olive oil, onion, tomato sauce, carrots, turnips, and shredded steak to the cooking liquid in the pot.
4. Stir in black pepper, sugar, and lemon juice to season the soup.
5. Cover the cabbage soup and cook on low heat for 1 ½ hour.
6. Serve warm.

Nutritions: *Calories: 212, Protein: 19g, Carbohydrates: 10g, Fat: 10g, Cholesterol: 60 Mg, Sodium: 242mg, Potassium: 388mg, Phosphorus: 160mg, Calcium: 46mg, Fiber: 2.1g*

242. GROUND BEEF SOUP

PREPARATION: 10 MIN **COOKING: 30 MIN** **SERVES: 4**

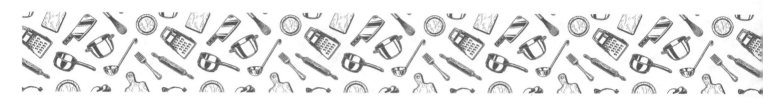

INGREDIENTS

- 1-pound lean ground beef
- ½ cup onion, chopped
- 2 teaspoons lemon-pepper seasoning blend
- 1 cup beef broth
- 2 cups of water
- 1/3 cup white rice, uncooked
- 3 cups frozen mixed vegetables
- 1 tablespoon sour cream

DIRECTIONS

1. Spray a saucepan with cooking oil and place it over medium heat.
2. Toss in onion and ground beef, then sauté until brown.
3. Stir in broth and rest of the ingredients, then boil it.
4. Reduce heat to a simmer, then cover the soup to cook for 30 minutes.
5. Garnish with sour cream.
6. Enjoy.

Nutritions: Calories: 223, Protein: 20g, Carbohydrates: 20g, Fat: 8g, Cholesterol: 52mg, Sodium: 170mg, Potassium: 448mg, Phosphorus: 210mg, Calcium: 43mg, Fiber: 4.3g

243. SHRIMP AND CRAB GUMBO

PREPARATION: 10 MIN

COOKING: 15 MIN

SERVES: 4

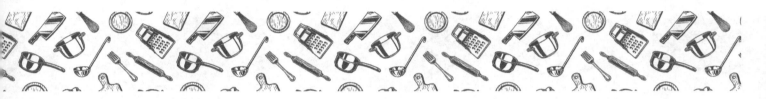

INGREDIENTS

- 1 cup bell pepper, chopped
- 1 ½ cups onion, chopped
- 1 garlic clove, chopped
- ¼ cup celery leaves, chopped
- 1 cup green onion tops
- ¼ cup fresh parsley, chopped
- 4 tablespoons canola oil
- 6 tablespoons all-purpose white flour
- 3 cups of water
- 4 cups chicken broth
- 8 ounces shrimp, uncooked
- 6 ounces crab meat
- ¼ teaspoon black pepper
- 1 teaspoon hot sauce
- 3 cups cooked rice

DIRECTIONS

1. Prepare the roux in a suitably-sized pan by heating oil in it.
2. Stir in flour and sauté until it changes its color.
3. Pour in 1 cup water, then add onion, garlic, celery leaves, and bell pepper.
4. Cover the roux mixture and cook on low heat until the veggies turn soft.
5. Add 2 cups water and 4 cups broth, then mix again.
6. Continue cooking it for 5 minutes then add crab meat and shrimp.
7. Cook for 10 minutes then and parsley and green onion.
8. Continue cooking for 5 minutes then garnish with black pepper and hot sauce.
9. Serve warm with rice.

Nutritions: *calories: 328, protein: 22g, carbohydrates: 34g, fat: 11g, cholesterol: 86mg, sodium: 328mg, potassium: 368mg, phosphorus: 221mg, calcium: 79mg, fiber: 1.4g*

244. TANGY TURKEY SOUP

PREPARATION: 10 MIN

COOKING: 68 MIN

SERVES: 4

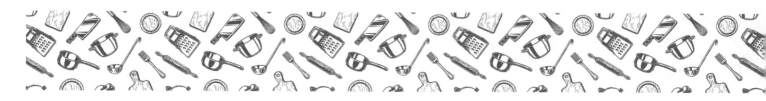

INGREDIENTS

- 1 cup carrots, chopped
- 1 cup celery, chopped
- 1 cup green bell pepper, chopped
- 1 cup yellow onion, chopped
- ½ cup fresh tomato, chopped
- ½ cup fresh parsley, chopped
- 2 garlic cloves, chopped
- 1 cup mushrooms, sliced
- 2 cups zucchini, sliced
- 1 tablespoon olive oil
- 1-pound turkey breast, skinless, cubed
- ½ teaspoon black pepper
- ½ cup dry white wine
- 4 cups chicken broth
- 1 teaspoon dried thyme
- 1 bay leaf
- ¼ teaspoon crushed red pepper
- 3 cups white rice, cooked
- 3 tablespoons lemon juice

DIRECTIONS

1. Place a suitably-sized stockpot over medium heat and oil to heat.
2. Toss in turkey, and black pepper, then sauté for 10 minutes.
3. Stir in green bell pepper, onion, celery, and carrots, then sauté for 8 minutes.
4. Add garlic, tomato, and wine then cook for 2 minutes.
5. Stir in bay leaf, thyme, broth, and red pepper then cook for 30 minutes on a simmer.
6. Add zucchini, mushrooms, parsley, and rice to the soup then continue cooking for 15 minutes.
7. Serve warm with lemon juice on top.

Nutritions: Calories: 215, Protein: 20g, Carbohydrates: 22g, Fat: 6g, Cholesterol: 24mg, Sodium: 128mg, Potassium: 528mg, Phosphorus: 197mg, Calcium: 54mg, Fiber: 2.4g

245. SPAGHETTI SQUASH & YELLOW BELL-PEPPER SOUP

PREPARATION: 10 MIN

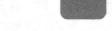

COOKING: 45 MIN

SERVES: 4

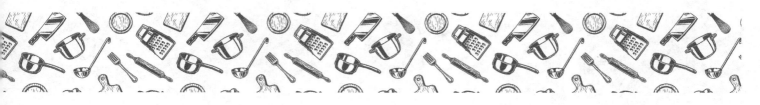

INGREDIENTS

- 2 diced yellow bell peppers
- 2 chopped large garlic cloves
- 1 peeled and cubed spaghetti squash
- 1 quartered and sliced onion
- 1 tablespoon dried thyme
- 1 tablespoon coconut oil
- 1 teaspoon curry powder
- 4 cups water

DIRECTIONS

1. Heat the oil before sweating the onions and garlic for 3-4 minutes.
2. Sprinkle over the curry powder.
3. Add in the stock and then bring to a boil over a high heat before adding the squash, pepper and thyme.
4. Turn down the heat, cover and allow to simmer for 25-30 minutes.
5. Continue to simmer until squash is soft if needed.
6. Allow to cool before blitzing in a blender/food processor until smooth.
7. Serve!

Nutritions: *Calories 103, Protein 2g, Carbs 17g, Fat 4g, Sodium (Na) 32mg, Potassium (K)365mg, Phosphorus 50mg*

246. RED PEPPER & BRIE SOUP

PREPARATION: 10 MIN

COOKING: 35 MIN

SERVES: 4

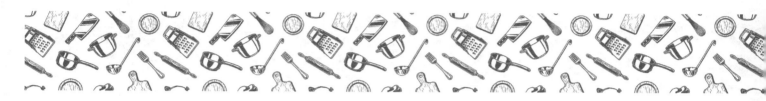

INGREDIENTS

- 1 teaspoon paprika
- 1 teaspoon cumin
- 1 chopped red onion
- 2 chopped garlic cloves
- ¼ cup crumbled brie
- 2 tablespoons. Extra virgin olive oil
- 4 chopped red bell peppers
- 4 cups water

DIRECTIONS

1. Sweat in the peppers & onion for 5 minutes.
2. Add the garlic cloves, cumin and paprika and sauté for 3-4 minutes.
3. Add the water and allow to boil before turning the heat down to simmer for 30 minutes.
4. And then remove it from the heat and then allow it to cool slightly.
5. Blend it until smooth after putting the mixture in a food processor.
6. Pour into serving bowls and add the crumbled brie to the top with a little black pepper.
7. Enjoy!

Nutritions: Calories 152, Protein 3g, Carbs 8g, Fat 11g, Sodium (Na) 66mg, Potassium (K) 270mg, Phosphorus 207mg

247. TURKEY & LEMON-GRASS SOUP

PREPARATION: 5 MIN

COOKING: 40 MIN

SERVES: 4

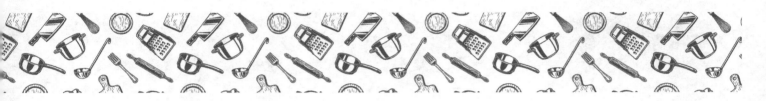

INGREDIENTS

- 1 fresh lime
- ¼ cup fresh basil leaves
- 1 tablespoon cilantro
- 1 cup canned and drained water chestnuts
- 1 tablespoon coconut oil
- 1 thumb-size minced ginger piece
- 2 chopped scallions
- 1 finely chopped green chili
- 4 ounce skinless and sliced turkey breasts
- 1 minced garlic clove, minced
- ½ finely sliced stick lemon-grass
- 1 chopped white onion, chopped
- 4 cups water

DIRECTIONS

1. Crush the lemon-grass, cilantro, chili, 1 tablespoon oil and basil leaves in a blender or pestle and mortar to form a paste.
2. Heat a large pan/wok with 1 tablespoon olive oil on high heat.
3. Sauté the onions, garlic and ginger until soft.
4. Add the turkey and brown each side for 4-5 minutes.
5. Add the broth and stir.
6. Now add the paste and stir.
7. Next add the water chestnuts, turn down the heat slightly and allow to simmer for 25-30 minutes or until turkey is thoroughly cooked through.
8. Serve hot with the green onion sprinkled over the top.

Nutritions: *Calories 123, Protein 10g, Carbs 12g, Fat 3g, Sodium (Na) 501mg, Potassium (K) 151mg, Phosphorus 110mg*

248. PAPRIKA PORK SOUP

PREPARATION: 5 MIN

COOKING: 35 MIN

SERVES: 2

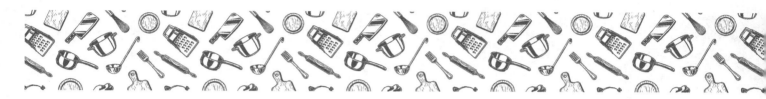

INGREDIENTS

- 4-ounce sliced pork loin
- 1 teaspoon black pepper
- 2 minced garlic cloves
- 1 cup baby spinach
- 3 cups water
- 1 tablespoon extra-virgin olive oil
- 1 chopped onion
- 1 tablespoon paprika

DIRECTIONS

1. Add in the oil, chopped onion and minced garlic.
2. Sauté for 5 minutes on low heat.
3. Add the pork slices to the onions and cook for 7-8 minutes or until browned.
4. Add the water to the pan and bring to a boil on high heat.
5. Stir in the spinach, reduce heat and simmer for a further 20 minutes or until pork is thoroughly cooked through.
6. Season with pepper to serve.

Nutritions: Calories 165, Protein 13g, Carbs 10g, Fat 9g, Sodium (Na) 269mg, Potassium (K) 486mg, Phosphorus 158mg

249. MEDITERRANEAN VEGETABLE SOUP

PREPARATION: 5 MIN

COOKING: 30 MIN

SERVES: 4

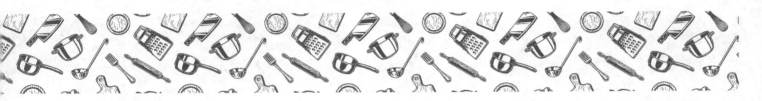

INGREDIENTS

- 1 tablespoon oregano
- 2 minced garlic cloves
- 1 teaspoon black pepper
- 1 diced zucchini
- 1 cup diced eggplant
- 4 cups water
- 1 diced red pepper
- 1 tablespoon extra-virgin olive oil
- 1 diced red onion

DIRECTIONS

1. Soak the vegetables in warm water prior to use.
2. Add in the oil, chopped onion and minced garlic.
3. Sweat for 5 minutes on low heat.
4. Add the other vegetables to the onions and cook for 7-8 minutes.
5. Add the stock to the pan and bring to a boil on high heat.
6. Stir in the herbs, reduce the heat, and simmer for a further 20 minutes or until thoroughly cooked through.
7. Season with pepper to serve.

Nutritions: *Calories 152, Protein 1g, Carbs 6g, Fat 3g, Sodium (Na) 3mg, Potassium (K) 229mg, Phosphorus 45mg*

250. TOFU SOUP

PREPARATION: 5 MIN

COOKING: 10 MIN

SERVES: 2

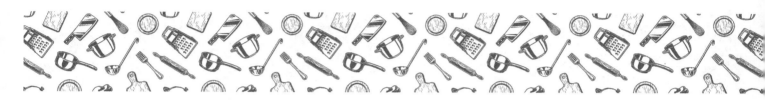

INGREDIENTS

- 1 tablespoon miso paste
- 1/8 cup cubed soft tofu
- 1 chopped green onion
- ¼ cup sliced shiitake mushrooms
- 3 cups renal stock
- 1 tablespoon soy sauce

DIRECTIONS

1. Take a saucepan, pour the stock into this pan and let it boil on high heat. Reduce heat to medium and let this stock simmer. Add mushrooms in this stock and cook for almost 3 minutes.
2. Take a bowl and mix soy sauce (reduced salt) and miso paste together in this bowl. Add this mixture and tofu in stock. Simmer for nearly 5 minutes and serve with chopped green onion.

Nutritions: Calories 129, Fat 7.8g, Sodium (Na) 484mg, Potassium (K) 435mg, Protein 11g, Carbs 5.5g, Phosphorus 73.2mg

251. ONION SOUP

PREPARATION: 15 MIN

COOKING: 45 MIN

SERVES: 6

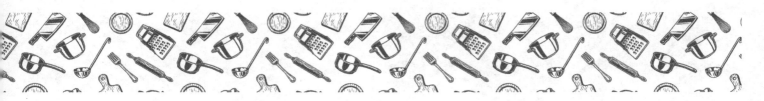

INGREDIENTS

- 2 tablespoons. Chicken stock
- 1 cup chopped shiitake mushrooms
- 1 tablespoon minced chives
- 3 teaspoons. Beef bouillon
- 1 teaspoon grated ginger root
- ½ chopped carrot
- 1 cup sliced portobello mushrooms
- 1 chopped onion
- ½ chopped celery stalk
- 2 quarts water
- ¼ teaspoon minced garlic

DIRECTIONS

1. Take a saucepan and combine carrot, onion, celery, garlic, mushrooms (some mushrooms) and ginger in this pan. Add water, beef bouillon and chicken stock in this pan. Put this pot on high heat and let it boil. Decrease flame to medium and cover this pan to cook for almost 45 minutes.
2. Put all remaining mushrooms in one separate pot. Once the boiling mixture is completely done, put one strainer over this new bowl with mushrooms and strain cooked soup in this pot over mushrooms. Discard solid-strained materials.
3. Serve delicious broth with yummy mushrooms in small bowls and sprinkle chives over each bowl.

Nutritions: *Calories 22, Fat 0g, Sodium (Na) 602.3mg, Potassium (K) 54.1mg, Carbs 4.9g, Protein 0.6g, Phosphorus 15.8mg*

252. STEAKHOUSE SOUP

PREPARATION: 15 MIN

COOKING: 25 MIN

SERVES: 4

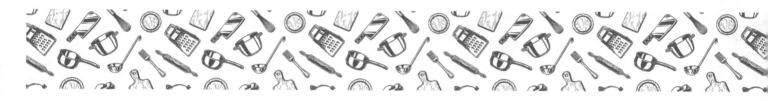

INGREDIENTS

- 2 tablespoons. Soy sauce
- 2 boneless and cubed chicken breasts.
- ¼ pound halved and trimmed snow peas
- 1 tablespoon minced ginger root
- 1 minced garlic clove
- 1 cup water
- 2 chopped green onions
- 3 cups chicken stock
- 1 chopped carrot
- 3 sliced mushrooms

DIRECTIONS

1. Take a pot and combine ginger, water, chicken stock, soy sauce (reduced salt) and garlic in this pot. Let them boil on medium heat, mix in chicken pieces, and let them simmer on low heat for almost 15 minutes to tender chicken.
2. Stir in carrot and snow peas and simmer for almost 5 minutes. Add mushrooms in this blend and continue cooking to tender vegetables for nearly 3 minutes. Mix in the chopped onion and serve hot.

Nutritions: Calories 319, Carbs 14g, Fat 15g, Potassium (K) 225mg, Protein 29g, Sodium (Na) 389mg, Phosphorous 190mg

253. CHINESE-STYLE BEEF STEW

PREPARATION: 15 MIN

COOKING: 6-8 H

SERVES: 6

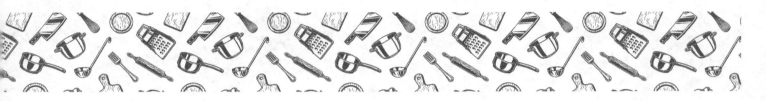

INGREDIENTS

- 2 medium carrots
- 2 green onions
- 2 celery stalks
- 1 medium green bell pepper, sliced
- 1 garlic clove
- 8 ounce of canned bean sprouts
- 8 ounce of canned water chestnuts
- 2 tablespoon of coconut oil
- 12ounce lean casserole beef, cut into cubes
- ½ cup low-sodium beef stock
- 1 tablespoon brown sugar
- 1/4 cup white wine vinegar
- 1 red chili, finely diced
- 1 ½ cups of water
- 3 cups cooked white rice

DIRECTIONS

1. Slice the carrots, green onions, celery and green pepper.
2. Crush the garlic. (hint: use the flat edge of a knife to do this easily.)
3. Rinse and slice the bamboo shoots and water chestnuts.
4. Heat the coconut oil and just brown the beef all over.
5. Transfer the beef to the slow cooker.
6. Add all the ingredients except the water.
7. Stir, it and then cover and cook on low for 6 to 8 hours.
8. Turn the slow cooker up to high.
9. Add the cold water to the slow cooker.
10. Stir it in to make it smooth, and leave the cooker lid slightly open.
11. Cook for a further 15 minutes.
12. Serve your dish over a bed of rice.

Nutritions: *Calories: 267, Protein: 14g, Carbohydrates: 31g, Fat: 9g, Cholesterol: 35mg, Sodium: 166mg, Potassium: 319mg, Phosphorus: 148mg, Calcium: 41mg, Fiber: 3g*

254. STUFFED BELL PEPPER SOUP

PREPARATION: 5 MIN

COOKING: 20 MIN

SERVES: 2

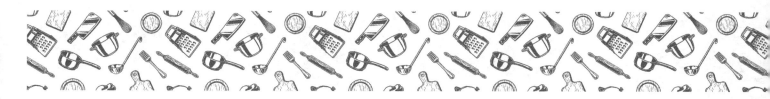

INGREDIENTS

- Chicken broth, low-sodium – 2 cups
- Bell pepper, red, diced – 1
- Garlic, minced – 4 cloves
- Onion, diced - .5 cup
- Ground turkey – 4 ounces
- Olive oil – 2 teaspoons
- Italian seasoning – 1 teaspoon
- White rice, cooked – 1 cup
- Parsley, fresh, chopped – 1 tablespoon

DIRECTIONS

1. Cook the ground turkey with the onion, olive oil, and garlic until the turkey is fully cooked and no pink is remaining about five to seven minutes.
2. Add the black pepper, italian seasoning, and bell pepper to the soup pot, allowing it to cook for three more minutes.
3. Into the pot, pour the low-sodium chicken broth, simmer the soup for fifteen minutes, until the bell peppers are tender. Stir in the cooked rice and parsley before serving.

Nutritions: Calories 283, Protein Grams: 16, Phosphorus Milligrams: 183, Potassium Milligrams: 369, Sodium Milligrams: 85, Fat Grams: 9, Total Carbohydrates Grams: 32, Net Carbohydrates Grams: 30

255. SALMON CHOWDER

PREPARATION: 20 MIN   COOKING: 4 H   SERVES: 2

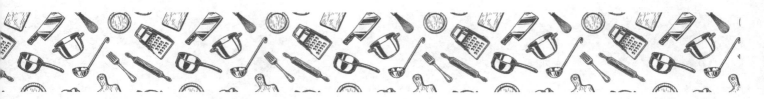

INGREDIENTS

- 3 pounds salmon fillets, sliced into manageable pieces
- 1 1/2 cups onion, chopped
- 2 potatoes, cubed – limit this
- 3 cups water
- 1/3 teaspoon pepper
- 18-ounce evaporated milk, non-fat

DIRECTIONS

1. Put together onion, salmon, potatoes, and pepper in the slow cooker. Pour water
2. Cover and cook for 8 hours on low. Secure the lid.
3. Cooking cycle, turn off the heat. Adjust seasoning according to your preferred taste.
4. Stir in milk. Cover and cook for another 30 minutes. Serve right away.

Nutritions: *Protein: 33.8g, Potassium: 204.3mg, Sodium: 183.5mg*

256. BEEF STEW PASTA

PREPARATION: 15 MIN

COOKING: 8 H

SERVES: 2

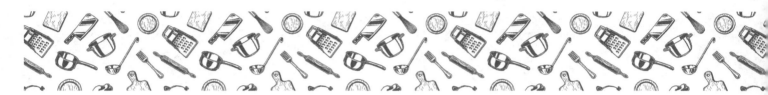

INGREDIENTS

- 1 tablespoon olive oil
- 3/4-pound beef round roast, sliced into bite-sized pieces
- 1/2 cup onion, chopped
- 1/2 cup carrots, chopped
- 1/2 cup celery, chopped
- 2 cups beef broth, no salt
- 1/2 teaspoon oregano
- 1/4 cup red wine
- 1/4 teaspoon thyme
- 1/4 teaspoon black pepper
- 2 small tomatoes, diced – limit this
- 1/4 cup whole wheat pasta

DIRECTIONS

1. Pour olive oil into non-stick skillet. Cook beef round roast, in batches, for 5 minutes or until browned all over. Transfer meat to the slow cooker.
2. Add in onion, tomatoes, carrots, celery, beef broth, oregano, red wine, thyme, black pepper, and pasta. Stir mixture well.
3. Cover and cook for 8 to 9 hours on low. Secure the lid.
4. After the 9-hour cooking cycle, turn off the heat. Adjust seasoning according to your preferred taste.
5. To serve, place pasta into plates. Pour sauce all over.

Nutritions: Protein: 12.8g, Potassium: 128.5mg, Sodium: 95.8mg

257. ITALIAN CHICKEN STEW

PREPARATION: 20 MIN

COOKING: 8 H

SERVES: 1

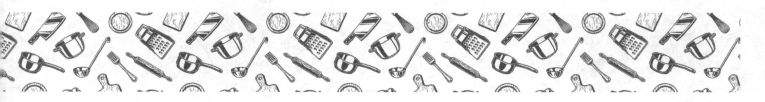

INGREDIENTS

- 1/2-pound chicken breast, boneless, skinless, cubed
- 1/3 cup celery, chopped
- 1/2 cup carrot, chopped
- 1/2 cup onion, chopped
- 2 ounce any kind of mushrooms, sliced
- 1/4 teaspoon dill weed
- 1/2 teaspoon italian seasoning
- 1/4 teaspoon basil
- 1/4 teaspoon black pepper
- 1 tomato, diced – limit this

DIRECTIONS

1. Place chicken breast cubes into the slow cooker.
2. Add in onion, carrot, italian seasoning, mushrooms, celery, basil, dill weed, and black pepper. Add in diced tomatoes. Mix well.
3. Cover and cook for 8 to 9 hours on low. Secure the lid.
4. After 9hr of cooking, turn off the heat. Adjust seasoning according to your preferred taste.
5. Serve warm.

Nutritions: *Protein: 29.9g, Potassium: 89.6mg, Sodium: 56.3mg*

258. TURKEY PASTA STEW

PREPARATION: 10 MIN

COOKING: 8 H

SERVES: 1

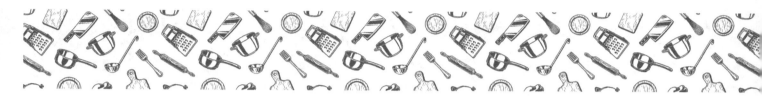

INGREDIENTS

- 1/2-pound ground turkey
- 1/2 cup carrots, sliced
- 1/2 fennel bulb, chopped
- 1/4 cup celery, sliced
- 1 cup chicken broth, low sodium
- 1/3 teaspoon garlic, minced
- 1/2 teaspoon oregano
- 1/2 teaspoon basil
- 1/2 cup shell pasta, uncooked
- 1 cup navy beans, unsalted, cooked

DIRECTIONS

1. Cook turkey in a non-stick skillet set over medium heat until browned on all sides. Transfer to the slow cooker.
2. Add in garlic, carrots, chicken broth, navy beans, basil celery, pasta, oregano, and fennel. Stir well to combine.
3. Cover and cook for 8 to 9 hours on low. Secure the lid.
4. After the 8-hour cooking cycle, turn off the heat. Adjust seasoning according to your preferred taste. Serve warm.

Nutritions: Protein: 18.8g, Potassium: 84.6mg, Sodium: 68.5mg

259. ONE-POT CHICKEN PIE STEW

PREPARATION: 15 MIN

COOKING: 1 H 15 MIN

SERVES: 8

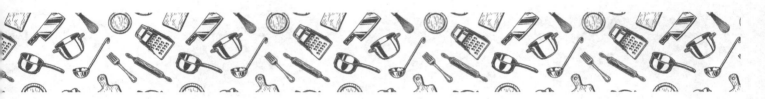

INGREDIENTS

- Fresh chicken breast (skinless and boneless) – 1½ pounds
- Low-sodium chicken stock – 2 cups
- Canola oil – ¼ cup
- Flour – ½ cup
- Fresh carrots (diced) – ½ cup
- Fresh onions (diced) – ½ cup
- Fresh celery (diced) – ¼ cup
- Black pepper – ½ teaspoon
- Italian seasoning (sodium-free) – 1 tablespoon
- Low-sodium better than bouillon® chicken base – 2 teaspoons
- Frozen sweet peas (thawed) – ½ cup
- Heavy cream – ½ cup
- Frozen piecrust (cooked, broken into bite-sized pieces) – 1
- Cheddar cheese (low-fat) – 1 cup

DIRECTIONS

1. Start by pounding the chicken to tenderize it. Cut into small equal-sized cubes.
2. Place it over a medium-high flame. Add in the stock and the chicken. Cook for about 30 minutes.
3. Add in the flour and oil, while the chicken is cooking, mix well to combine.
4. Stir the flour and oil mixture into the broth mixture. Keep stirring until the chicken broth starts to thicken.
5. Reduce the flame to low and cook for another 15 minutes.
6. Now add in the carrots, celery, onions, italian seasoning, bouillon, and black pepper. Cook for another 15 minutes.
7. Add in the cream and peas after turning off the flame. Keep stirring to mix well.
8. Transfer into soup mugs and top with the cheese and broken pie crust pieces.

Nutritions: *protein 26g, carbohydrates 22g, fat 21g, cholesterol 82mg, sodium 424mg, potassium 209mg, phosphorus 290mg, calcium 88mg, fiber 2g*

260. CAULIFLOWER AND ASPARAGUS TORTILLA

PREPARATION: 10 MIN

COOKING: 30 MIN

SERVES: 4

INGREDIENTS

- Asparagus – 2 cups
- Cauliflower – 2 cups
- Olive oil – 2 teaspoons
- Onion – 1½ cups
- Garlic – 1 clove
- Liquid egg substitute (low-cholesterol) – 1 cup
- Fresh parsley (finely chopped) – 2 tablespoons
- Salt – ¼ teaspoon
- Pepper (freshly ground) – ½ teaspoon
- Dried thyme leaves (crushed) – ¼ teaspoon
- Ground nutmeg – ¼ teaspoon

DIRECTIONS

1. Start by chopping the asparagus and cauliflower into 1-inch pieces. Take the onion and chop it finely. Also, mince the garlic clove.
2. Take a microwave-safe bowl and place the chopped cauliflower and asparagus pieces into it. Add in 1 tablespoon of water and cover the dish.
3. After that, drain any excess water and set aside.
4. Microwave them for about 4-5 minutes. Make sure the veggies are slightly tender.
5. Place a saucepan over a high flame and pour the oil into it. Once heated, toss in the finely chopped onions.
6. Sauté the onions for about 6-7 minutes. Add in the minced garlic and sauté for 1 more minute.
7. Toss in the cauliflower, asparagus, egg substitute, salt, thyme, parsley, and nutmeg. Arrange them well over the egg substitute base.
8. Cover the saucepan, and cook for about 15 minutes in low heat.
9. Use a butter knife to loosen the edges of the prepared tortilla.
10. Take a microwave-safe serving platter and heat it for about 30-40 seconds.
11. Invert the tortilla onto the heated serving platter. Serve hot!

Nutritions: Protein 9g, Fat 3g, Carbohydrates 9g, Sodium 248mg, Cholesterol 0mg, Potassium 472mg, Calcium 68mg, Phosphorus 97mg, Fiber 3.88g

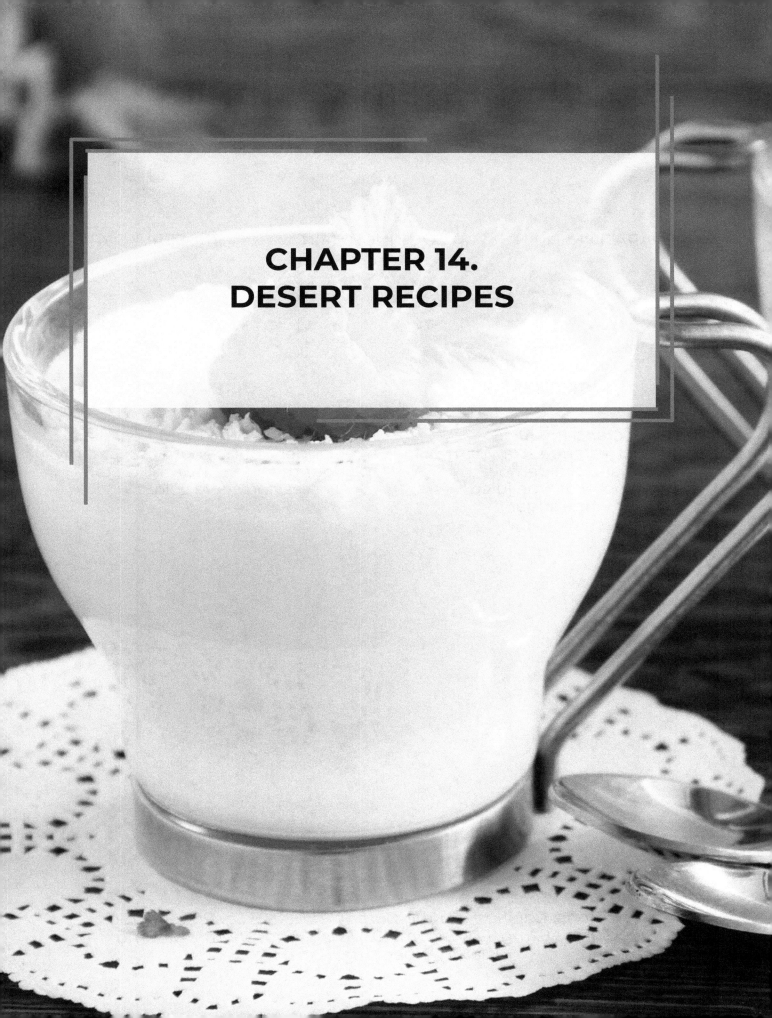

CHAPTER 14.
DESERT RECIPES

261. DESSERT COCKTAIL

PREPARATION: 1 MIN

COOKING: 0 MIN

SERVES: 4

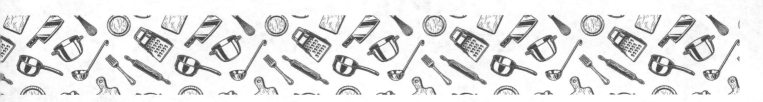

INGREDIENTS

- 1 cup of cranberry juice
- 1 cup of fresh ripe strawberries, washed and hull removed
- 2 tablespoon of lime juice
- ¼ cup of white sugar
- 8 ice cubes

DIRECTIONS

1. Combine all the ingredients in a blender until smooth and creamy.
2. Pour the liquid into chilled tall glasses and serve cold.

Nutritions: *Calories: 92 Kcal, Carbohydrate: 23.5g, Protein: 0.5g, Sodium: 3.62mg, Potassium: 103.78mg, Phosphorus: 17.86mg, Dietary Fiber: 0.8g, Fat: 0.17g*

262. BAKED EGG CUSTARD

PREPARATION: 15 MIN

COOKING: 30 MIN

SERVES: 4

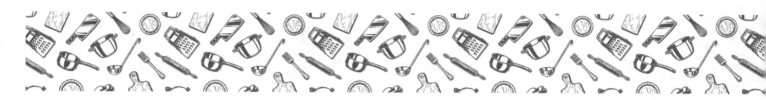

INGREDIENTS

- 2 medium eggs, at room temperature
- ¼ cup of semi-skimmed milk
- 3 tablespoons of white sugar
- ½ teaspoon of nutmeg
- 1 teaspoon of vanilla extract

DIRECTIONS

1. Preheat your oven at 375 f/180c
2. Mix all the ingredients in a mixing bowl and beat with a hand mixer for a few seconds until creamy and uniform.
3. Pour the mixture into lightly greased muffin tins.
4. Bake for 25-30 minutes or until the knife, you place inside, comes out clean.

Nutritions: Calories: 96.56 Kcal, Carbohydrate: 10.5g, Protein: 3.5g, Sodium: 37.75mg, Potassium: 58.19mg, Phosphorus: 58.76mg, Dietary Fiber: 0.06g, Fat: 2.91g

263. GUMDROP COOKIES

PREPARATION: 15 MIN

COOKING: 12 MIN

SERVES: 25

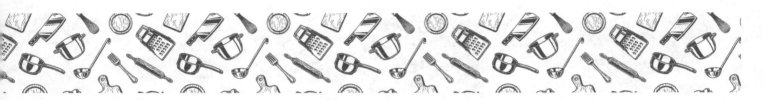

INGREDIENTS

- ½ cup of spreadable unsalted butter
- 1 medium egg
- 1 cup of brown sugar
- 1 2/3 cups of all-purpose flour, sifted
- ¼ cup of milk
- 1 teaspoon vanilla
- 1 teaspoon of baking powder
- 15 large gumdrops, chopped finely

DIRECTIONS

1. Preheat the oven at 400f/195c.
2. Combine the sugar, butter and egg until creamy.
3. Add the milk and vanilla and stir well.
4. Combine the flour with the baking powder in a different bowl. Incorporate to the sugar, butter mixture, and stir.
5. Add the gumdrops and place the mixture in the fridge for half an hour.
6. Drop the dough with tablespoonful into a lightly greased baking or cookie sheet.
7. Bake for 10-12 minutes or until golden brown in color.

Nutritions: *Calories: 102.17 Kcal, Carbohydrate: 16.5g, Protein: 0.86g, Sodium: 23.42mg, Potassium: 45mg, Phosphorus: 32.15mg, Dietary Fiber: 0.13g, Fat: 4g*

264. POUND CAKE WITH PINEAPPLE

PREPARATION: 10 MIN

COOKING: 50 MIN

SERVES: 24

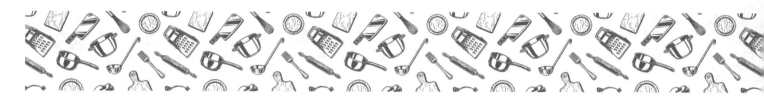

INGREDIENTS

- 3 cups of all-purpose flour, sifted
- 3 cups of sugar
- 1 ½ cups of butter
- 6 whole eggs and 3 egg whites
- 1 teaspoon of vanilla extract
- 1 10. Ounce can of pineapple chunks, rinsed and crushed (keep juice aside).

For glaze:
- 1 cup of sugar
- 1 stick of unsalted butter or margarine
- Reserved juice from the pineapple

DIRECTIONS

1. Preheat the oven at 350f/180c.
2. Beat the sugar and the butter with a hand mixer until creamy and smooth.
3. Slowly add the eggs (one or two every time) and stir well after pouring each egg.
4. Add the vanilla extract, follow up with the flour and stir well.
5. Add the drained and chopped pineapple.
6. Pour the mixture into a greased cake tin and bake for 45-50 minutes.
7. In a small saucepan, combine the sugar with the butter and pineapple juice. Stir every few seconds and bring to boil. Cook until you get a creamy to thick glaze consistency.
8. Pour the glaze over the cake while still hot.
9. Let cook for at least 10 seconds and serve.

Nutritions: Calories: 407.4 Kcal, Carbohydrate: 79g, Protein: 4.25g, Sodium: 118.97mg, Potassium: 180.32mg, Phosphorus: 66.37mg, Dietary Fiber: 2.25g, Fat: 16.48g

265. APPLE CRUNCH PIE

PREPARATION: 10 MIN

COOKING: 35 MIN

SERVES: 8

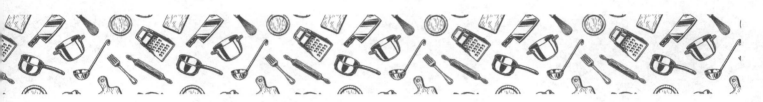

INGREDIENTS

- 4 large tart apples, peeled, seeded and sliced
- ½ cup of white all-purpose flour
- 1/3 cup margarine
- 1 cup of sugar
- ¾ cup of rolled oat flakes
- ½ teaspoon of ground nutmeg

DIRECTIONS

1. Preheat the oven to 375f/180c.
2. Place the apples over a lightly greased square pan (around 7 inches).
3. Mix the rest of the ingredients in a medium bowl with and spread the batter over the apples.
4. Bake for 30-35 minutes or until the top crust has gotten golden brown.
5. Serve hot.

Nutritions: *Calories: 261.9 Kcal, Carbohydrate: 47.2g, Protein: 1.5g, Sodium: 81mg, Potassium: 123.74mg, Phosphorus: 35.27mg, Dietary Fiber: 2.81g, Fat: 7.99g*

266. SPICED PEACHES

PREPARATION: 5 MIN

COOKING: 10 MIN

SERVES: 2

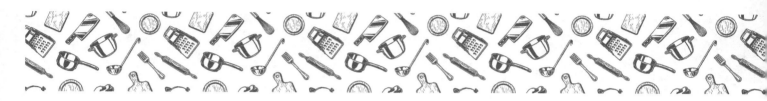

INGREDIENTS

- Canned peaches with juices – 1 cup
- Cornstarch – ½ teaspoon
- Ground cloves – 1 teaspoon
- Ground cinnamon – 1 teaspoon
- Ground nutmeg – 1 teaspoon
- Zest of ½ lemon
- Water – ½ cup

DIRECTIONS

1. Drain peaches.
2. Combine cinnamon, cornstarch, nutmeg, ground cloves, and lemon zest in a pan on the stove.
3. Heat on a medium heat and add peaches.
4. Bring to a boil, reduce the heat and simmer for 10 minutes.
5. Serve.

Nutritions: Calories: 70, Fat: 0,G Carb: 14g, Phosphorus: 23mg, Potassium: 176mg, Sodium: 3mg, Protein: 1g

267. PUMPKIN CHEESECAKE BAR

PREPARATION: 10 MIN

COOKING: 50 MIN

SERVES: 4

INGREDIENTS

- Unsalted butter – 2 ½ tablespoons.
- Cream cheese – 4 ounces
- All-purpose white flour – ½ cup
- Golden brown sugar – 3 tablespoons.
- Granulated sugar – ¼ cup
- Pureed pumpkin – ½ cup
- Egg whites - 2
- Ground cinnamon – 1 teaspoon
- Ground nutmeg – 1 teaspoon
- Vanilla extract – 1 teaspoon

DIRECTIONS

1. Preheat the oven to 350f.
2. Mix flour and brown sugar in a bowl.
3. Mix in the butter to form 'breadcrumbs.
4. Place ¾ of this mixture in a dish.
5. Bake in the oven for 15 minutes. Remove and cool.
6. Lightly whisk the egg and fold in the cream cheese, sugar, pumpkin, cinnamon, nutmeg and vanilla until smooth.
7. Pour this mixture over the oven-baked base and sprinkle with the rest of the breadcrumbs from earlier.
8. Bake in the oven for 30 to 35 minutes more.
9. Cool, slice and serve.

Nutritions: *Calories: 248, Fat: 13g, Carb: 33g, Phosphorus: 67mg, Potassium: 96mg, Sodium: 146mg, Protein: 4g*

268. BLUEBERRY MINI MUFFINS

PREPARATION: 10 MIN

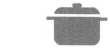

COOKING: 35 MIN

SERVES: 4

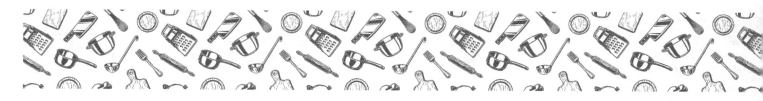

INGREDIENTS

- Egg whites – 3
- All-purpose white flour – ¼ cup
- Coconut flour – 1 tablespoon
- Baking soda – 1 teaspoon
- Nutmeg – 1 tablespoon grated
- Vanilla extract – 1 teaspoon
- Stevia – 1 teaspoon
- Fresh blueberries – ¼ cup

DIRECTIONS

1. Preheat the oven to 325f.
2. Mix all the ingredients in a bowl.
3. Divide the batter into 4 and spoon into a lightly oiled muffin tin.
4. Bake in the oven for 15 to 20 minutes or until cooked through.
5. Cool and serve.

Nutritions: Calories: 62, Fat: 0g, Carb: 9g, Phosphorus: 103mg, Potassium: 65mg, Sodium: 62mg, Protein: 4g

269. VANILLA CUSTARD

PREPARATION: 7 MIN

COOKING: 10 MIN

SERVES: 10

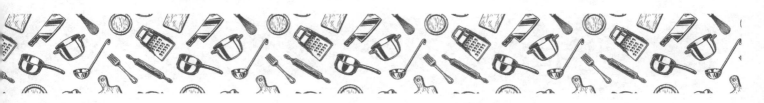

INGREDIENTS

- Egg – 1
- Vanilla – 1/8 teaspoon
- Nutmeg – 1/8 teaspoon
- Almond milk – ½ cup
- Stevia - 2 tablespoon

DIRECTIONS

1. Scald the milk then let it cool slightly.
2. Break the egg into a bowl and beat it with the nutmeg.
3. Add the scalded milk, the vanilla, and the sweetener to taste. Mix well.
4. Place the bowl in a baking pan filled with ½ deep of water.
5. Bake for 30 minutes at 325f.
6. Serve.

Nutritions: *Calories: 167.3, Fat: 9g, Carb: 11g, Phosphorus: 205mg, Potassium: 249mg, Sodium: 124mg, Protein: 10g*

270. CHOCOLATE CHIP COOKIES

PREPARATION: 7 MIN

COOKING: 10 MIN

SERVES: 10

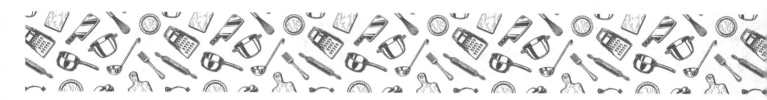

INGREDIENTS

- Semi-sweet chocolate chips – ½ cup
- Baking soda – ½ teaspoon
- Vanilla – ½ teaspoon
- Egg – 1
- Flour – 1 cup
- Margarine – ½ cup
- Stevia – 4 teaspoons

DIRECTIONS

1. Sift the dry ingredients.
2. Cream the margarine, stevia, vanilla and egg with a whisk.
3. Add flour mixture and beat well.
4. Stir in the chocolate chips, then drop teaspoonfuls of the mixture over a greased baking sheet.
5. Bake the cookies for about 10 minutes at 375f.
6. Cool and serve.

Nutritions: Calories: 106.2, Fat: 7g, Carb: 8.9g, Phosphorus: 19mg, Potassium: 28mg, Sodium: 98mg, Protein: 1.5g

271. LEMON MOUSSE

PREPARATION: 10 MIN + CHILL

COOKING: 10 MIN

SERVES: 4

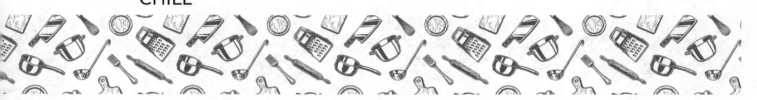

INGREDIENTS

- 1 cup coconut cream
- 8 ounces cream cheese, soft
- ¼ cup fresh lemon juice
- 3 pinches salt
- 1 teaspoon lemon liquid stevia

DIRECTIONS

1. Preheat your oven to 350 °f
2. Grease a ramekin with butter
3. Beat cream, cream cheese, fresh lemon juice, salt and lemon liquid stevia in a mixer
4. Pour batter into ramekin
5. Bake for 10 minutes, then transfer the mousse to a serving glass
6. Let it chill for 2 hours and serve
7. Enjoy!

Nutritions: *Calories: 395, Fat: 31g, Carbohydrates: 3g, Protein: 5g*

272. JALAPENO CRISP

PREPARATION: 10 MIN

COOKING: 1 H 15 MIN

SERVES: 20

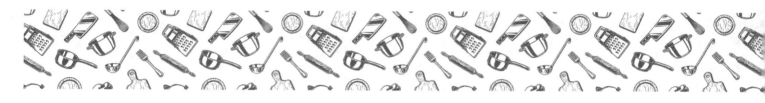

INGREDIENTS

- 1 cup sesame seeds
- 1 cup sunflower seeds
- 1 cup flaxseeds
- ½ cup hulled hemp seeds
- 3 tablespoons psyllium husk
- 1 teaspoon salt
- 1 teaspoon baking powder
- 2 cups of water

DIRECTIONS

1. Pre-heat your oven to 350 °f
2. Take your blender and add seeds, baking powder, salt, and psyllium husk
3. Blend well until a sand-like texture appears
4. Stir in water and mix until a batter form
5. Allow the batter to rest for 10 minutes until a dough-like thick mixture forms
6. Pour the dough onto a cookie sheet lined with parchment paper
7. Spread it evenly, making sure that it has a thickness of ¼ inch thick all around
8. Bake for 75 minutes in your oven
9. Remove and cut into 20 spices
10. Allow them to cool for 30 minutes and enjoy!

Nutritions: calories: 156, fat: 13g, carbohydrates: 2g, protein: 5g

273. RASPBERRY POPSICLE

PREPARATION: 2 H

COOKING: 15 MIN

SERVES: 4

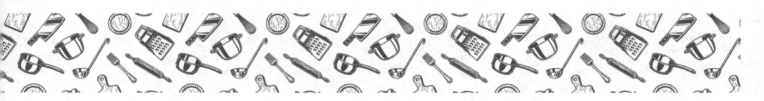

INGREDIENTS

- 1 ½ cups raspberries
- 2 cups of water

DIRECTIONS

1. Take a pan and fill it up with water
2. Add raspberries
3. Place it over medium heat and bring to water to a boil
4. Reduce the heat and simmer for 15 minutes
5. Remove heat and pour the mix into popsicle molds
6. Add a popsicle stick and let it chill for 2 hours
7. Serve and enjoy!

Nutritions: *Calories: 58, Fat: 0.4g, Carbohydrates: 0g, Protein: 1.4g*

274. EASY FUDGE

PREPARATION: 15 MIN + CHILL

COOKING: 5 MIN

SERVES: 25

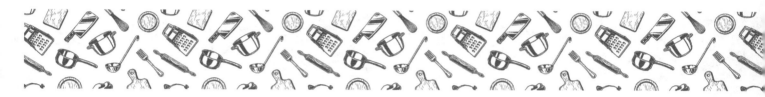

INGREDIENTS

- 1 ¾ cups of coconut butter
- 1 cup pumpkin puree
- 1 teaspoon ground cinnamon
- ¼ teaspoon ground nutmeg
- 1 tablespoon coconut oil

DIRECTIONS

1. Take an 8x8 inch square baking pan and line it with aluminum foil
2. Take a spoon and scoop out the coconut butter into a heated pan and allow the butter to melt
3. Keep stirring well and remove from the heat once fully melted
4. Add spices and pumpkin and keep straining until you have a grain-like texture
5. Add coconut oil and keep stirring to incorporate everything
6. Scoop the mixture into your baking pan and evenly distribute it
7. Place wax paper on top of the mixture and press gently to straighten the top
8. Remove the paper and discard
9. Allow it to chill for 1-2 hours
10. Once chilled, take it out and slice it up into pieces
11. Enjoy!

Nutritions: Calories: 120, Fat: 10g, Carbohydrates: 5g, Protein: 1.2g

275. COCONUT LOAF

PREPARATION: 15 MIN

COOKING: 40 MIN

SERVES: 4

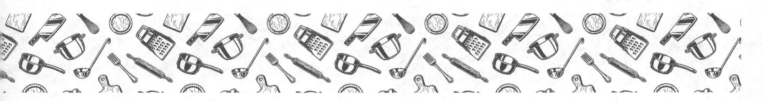

INGREDIENTS

- 1 ½ tablespoons coconut flour
- ¼ teaspoon baking powder
- 1/8 teaspoon salt
- 1 tablespoon coconut oil, melted
- 1 whole egg

DIRECTIONS

1. Preheat your oven to 350 °f
2. Add coconut flour, baking powder, salt
3. Add coconut oil, eggs and stir well until mixed
4. Leave the batter for several minutes
5. Pour half the batter onto the baking pan
6. Spread it to form a circle, repeat with remaining batter
7. Bake in the oven for 10 minutes
8. Once a golden-brown texture comes, let it cool and serve
9. Enjoy!

Nutritions: *Calories: 297, Fat: 14g, Carbohydrates: 15g, Protein: 15g*

276. CAULIFLOWER BAGEL

PREPARATION: 10 MIN

COOKING: 30 MIN

SERVES: 12

INGREDIENTS

- 1 large cauliflower, divided into florets and roughly chopped
- ¼ cup nutritional yeast
- ¼ cup almond flour
- ½ teaspoon garlic powder
- 1 ½ teaspoon fine sea salt
- 2 whole eggs
- 1 tablespoon sesame seeds

DIRECTIONS

1. Preheat your oven to 400 °f
2. Line a baking sheet with parchment paper, keep it on the side
3. Blend cauliflower in a food processor and transfer to a bowl
4. Add nutritional yeast, almond flour, garlic powder and salt to a bowl, mix
5. Take another bowl and whisk in eggs, add to cauliflower mix
6. Give the dough a stir
7. Incorporate the mix into the egg mix
8. Make balls from the dough, making a hole using your thumb into each ball
9. Arrange them on your prepped sheet, flattening them into bagel shapes
10. Sprinkle sesame seeds and bake for half an hour
11. Remove the oven and let them cool, enjoy!

Nutritions: Calories: 152, Fat: 10g, Carbohydrates: 4g, Protein: 4g

277. ALMOND CRACKERS

PREPARATION: 10 MIN **COOKING: 20 MIN** **SERVES: 40 CRACKERS**

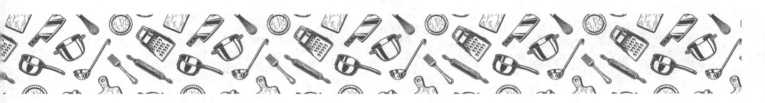

INGREDIENTS

- 1 cup almond flour
- ¼ teaspoon baking soda
- ¼ teaspoon salt
- 1/8 teaspoon black pepper
- 3 tablespoons sesame seeds
- 1 egg, beaten
- Salt and pepper to taste

DIRECTIONS

1. Preheat your oven to 350 °f
2. Line two baking sheets with parchment paper and keep them on the side
3. Mix the dry ingredients into a large bowl and add egg, mix well and form a dough
4. Divide dough into two balls
5. Roll out the dough. Do this between two pieces of parchment paper.
6. Cut into crackers and transfer them to prep a baking sheet
7. Bake for 15-20 minutes
8. Repeat this process until all the dough has been used up
9. Leave crackers to cool and serve
10. Enjoy!

Nutritions: *Calories: 302, Fat: 28g, Carbohydrates: 4g, Protein: 9g*

278. CASHEW AND ALMOND BUTTER

PREPARATION: 5 MIN

COOKING: 15 MIN

SERVES: 1 ½ CUPS

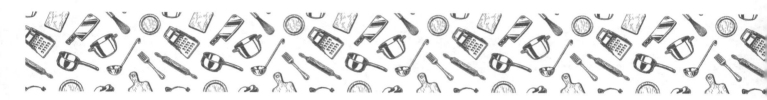

INGREDIENTS

- 1 cup almonds, blanched
- 1/3 cup cashew nuts
- 2 tablespoons coconut oil
- Salt as needed
- ½ teaspoon cinnamon

DIRECTIONS

1. Preheat your oven to 350 °f
2. Bake almonds and cashews for 12 minutes
3. Let them cool
4. Transfer to a food processor and add remaining ingredients
5. Add oil and keep blending until smooth
6. Serve and enjoy!

Nutritions: calories: 205, fat: 19g, protein: 2.8g

279. NUT AND CHIA MIX

PREPARATION: 10 MIN

COOKING: 0 MIN

SERVES: 1

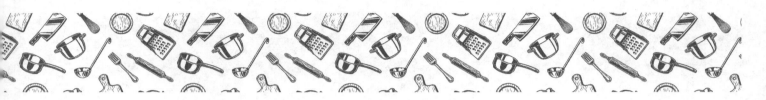

INGREDIENTS

- 1 tablespoon chia seeds
- 2 cups of water
- 1-ounce macadamia nuts
- 1-2 packets stevia, optional
- 1-ounce hazelnuts

DIRECTIONS

1. Add all the listed ingredients to a blender.
2. Blend on high until smooth and creamy.
3. Enjoy your smoothie.

Nutritions: *Calories: 452, Fat: 43g, Carbohydrates: 15g, Protein: 9g*

280. HEARTY CUCUMBER BITES

PREPARATION: 5 MIN   **COOKING: 0 MIN**   **SERVES: 4**

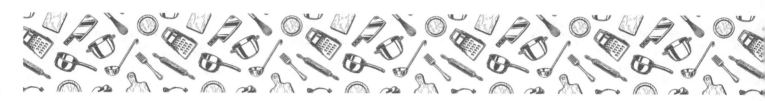

INGREDIENTS

- 1 (8 ounces) cream cheese container, low fat
- 1 tablespoon bell pepper, diced
- 1 tablespoon shallots, diced
- 1 tablespoon parsley, chopped
- 2 cucumbers
- Pepper to taste

DIRECTIONS

1. Take a bowl and add cream cheese, onion, pepper, parsley
2. Peel cucumbers and cut in half
3. Remove seeds and stuff with the cheese mix
4. Cut into bite-sized portions and enjoy!

Nutritions: Calories: 85, Fat: 4g, Carbohydrates: 2g, Protein: 3g

281. HEARTY ALMOND BREAD

PREPARATION: 15 MIN

COOKING: 60 MIN

SERVES: 8

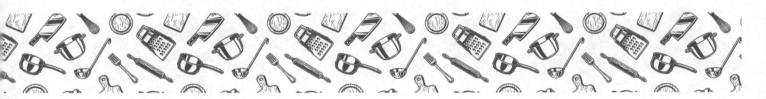

INGREDIENTS

- 3 cups almond flour
- 1 teaspoon baking soda
- 2 teaspoons baking powder
- ¼ teaspoon sunflower seeds
- ¼ cup almond milk
- ½ cup + 2 tablespoons olive oil
- 3 whole eggs

DIRECTIONS

1. Preheat your oven to 300 ° f
2. Take a 9x5 inch loaf pan and grease, keep it on the side
3. Add the listed ingredients to a bowl and pour the batter into the loaf pan
4. Bake for 60 minutes
5. Once baked, remove this from oven and let it cool
6. Slice and serve!

Nutritions: *Calories: 277, Fat: 21g, Carbohydrates: 7g, Protein: 10g*

282. MEDJOOL BALLS

PREPARATION: 5 MIN +20 MIN CHILL

COOKING: 2-3 MIN

SERVES: 4

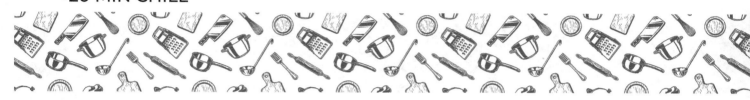

INGREDIENTS

- 3 cups Medrol dates, chopped
- 12 ounces brewed coffee
- 1 cup pecan, chopped
- ½ cup coconut, shredded
- ½ cup of cocoa powder

DIRECTIONS

1. Soak dates in warm coffee for 5 minutes
2. Remove dates from coffee and mash them, making a fine smooth mixture
3. Stir in the remaining ingredients (except cocoa powder) and form small balls out of the mixture
4. Coat with cocoa powder, serve and enjoy!

Nutritions: Calories: 265, Fat: 12g, Carbohydrates: 43g, Protein 3g

283. BLUEBERRY PUDDING

PREPARATION: 20 MIN

COOKING: 0 MIN

SERVES: 4

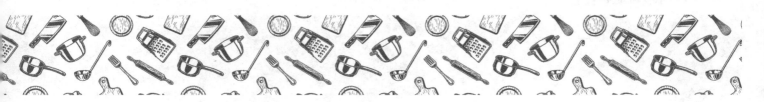

INGREDIENTS

- 2 cups of frozen blueberries
- 2 teaspoon of lime zest, grated freshly
- 20 drops of liquid stevia
- ½ teaspoon of fresh ginger, grated freshly
- 4 tablespoon of fresh lime juice
- 10 tablespoons of water

DIRECTIONS

1. Add all of the listed ingredients to a blender (except blueberries) and pulse the mixture well
2. Transfer the mix into small serving bowls and chill the bowls
3. Serve with a topping of blueberries
4. Enjoy!

Nutritions: *Calories: 166, Fat: 13g, Carbohydrates: 13g, Protein: 1.7g*

284. CHIA SEED PUMPKIN PUDDING

PREPARATION: 10-15 MIN /OVERNIGHT CHILL

COOKING: 50 MIN

SERVES: 4

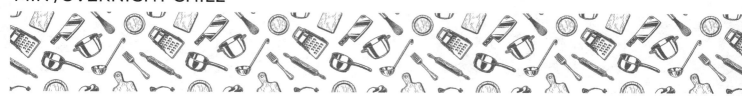

INGREDIENTS

- 1 cup maple syrup
- 2 teaspoons pumpkin spice
- 1 cup pumpkin puree
- 1 ¼ cup of almond milk
- ½ cup chia seeds

DIRECTIONS

1. Add all of the ingredients to a bowl and gently stir
2. Let it refrigerate overnight or for at least 15 minutes
3. Top with your desired ingredients such as blueberries, almonds, etcetera.
4. Serve and enjoy!

Nutritions: Calories: 230, Fat: 10g, Carbohydrates:22g, Protein: 11g

285. PARSLEY SOUFFLE

PREPARATION: 5 MIN

COOKING: 6 MIN

SERVES: 5

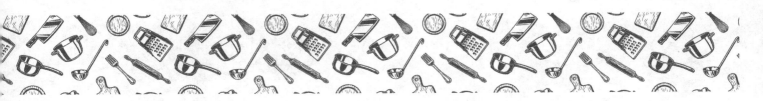

INGREDIENTS

- 2 whole eggs
- 1 fresh red chili pepper, chopped
- 2 tablespoons coconut cream
- 1 tablespoon fresh parsley, chopped
- Sunflower seeds to taste

DIRECTIONS

1. Preheat your oven to 390 °f
2. Almond butter two soufflé dishes
3. Add the ingredients to a blender and mix well
4. Divide batter into soufflé dishes and bake for 6 minutes
5. Serve and enjoy!

Nutritions: *Calories: 108, Fat: 9g, Carbohydrates: 9g, Protein: 6g*

286. ELEGANT VEGGIE TORTILLAS

PREPARATION: 30 MIN

COOKING: 15 MIN

SERVES: 12

INGREDIENTS

- 1½ cups of chopped broccoli florets
- 1½ cups of chopped cauliflower florets
- 1 tablespoon of water
- 2 teaspoon of canola oil
- 1½ cups of chopped onion
- 1 minced garlic clove
- 2 tablespoons of finely chopped fresh parsley
- 1 cup of low-cholesterol liquid egg substitute
- Freshly ground black pepper, to taste
- 4 (6-ounce) warmed corn tortillas

DIRECTIONS

1. In a microwave bowl, place broccoli, cauliflower and water and microwave, covered for about 3-5 minutes.
2. Remove from microwave and drain any liquid.
3. Heat oil on medium heat.
4. Add onion and sauté for about 4-5 minutes.
5. Add garlic and then sauté it for about 1 minute.
6. Stir in broccoli, cauliflower, parsley, egg substitute and black pepper.
7. Reduce the heat and it to simmer for about 10 minutes.
8. Remove from heat and keep aside to cool slightly.
9. Place broccoli mixture over ¼ of each tortilla.
10. Fold the outside edges inward and roll up like a burrito.
11. Secure each tortilla with toothpicks to secure the filling.
12. Cut each tortilla in half and serve.

Nutritions: Calories: 217, Fat: 3.3g, Carbs: 41g, Protein: 8.1g, Fiber: 6.3g, Potassium: 289mg, Sodium: 87mg

287. MUG CAKE POPPER

PREPARATION: 5 MIN

COOKING: 5 MIN

SERVES: 2

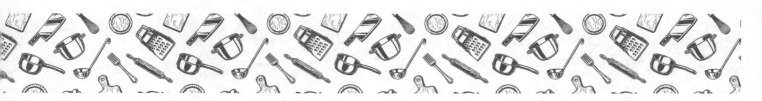

INGREDIENTS

- 2 tablespoons almond flour
- 1 tablespoon flaxseed meal
- 1 tablespoon almond butter
- 1 tablespoon cream cheese
- 1 large egg
- 1 bacon, cooked and sliced
- ½ jalapeno pepper
- ½ teaspoon baking powder
- ¼ teaspoon sunflower seeds

DIRECTIONS

1. Take a frying pan and place it over medium heat
2. Add sliced bacon and cook until they have a crispy texture
3. Take a microwave proof container and mix all of the listed ingredients (including cooked bacon), clean the sides
4. Microwave for 75 seconds making sure to put your microwave to high power
5. Take out the cup and slam it against a surface to take the cake out
6. Garnish with a bit of jalapeno and serve!

Nutritions: *Calories: 429, Fat: 38g, Carbohydrates: 6g, Protein: 16g*

288. CHEESECAKE BITES

PREPARATION: 10 MIN   **COOKING: 5 MIN**   **SERVES: 16**

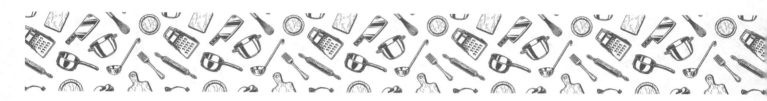

INGREDIENTS

- 8-ounce cream cheese
- 1/2 teaspoon vanilla
- 1/4 cup swerve

DIRECTIONS

1. Add all ingredients into the mixing bowl and blend until well combined.
2. Place bowl into the fridge for 1 hour.
3. Remove bowl from the fridge. Make small balls from cheese mixture and place them on a baking dish.
4. Serve and enjoy.

Nutritions: Calories 50, Fat 4.9g, Carbohydrates 0.4g, Sugar 0.1g, Protein 1.1g, Cholesterol 16mg

289. KETO MINT GINGER TEA

PREPARATION: 5 MIN

COOKING: 5 MIN

SERVES: 1

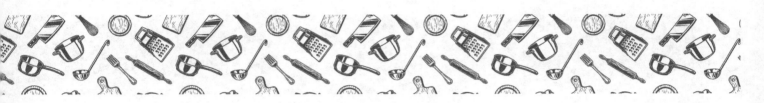

INGREDIENTS

- 1 1/2 tablespoon fresh mint leaves
- 1 cup of water
- 1/2 tablespoon fresh ginger, grated
- 1 teaspoon ground turmeric

DIRECTIONS

1. Add mint, ginger, and turmeric in boiling water.
2. Stir to turmeric dissolved.
3. Strain and serve.

Nutritions: *calories 19, fat 0.3g, carbohydrates 4g, sugar 0.3g, protein 0.5,g cholesterol 0mg*

290. KETO BROWNIE

PREPARATION: 10 MIN

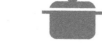

COOKING: 20 MIN

SERVES: 4

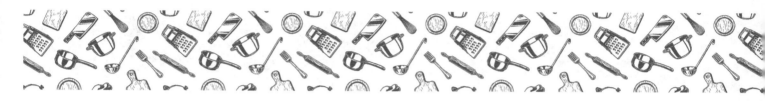

INGREDIENTS

- 2 tablespoon unsweetened cocoa powder
- 1/2 cup almond butter, melted
- 1 cup banana, overripe & mashed
- 1 scoop vanilla protein powder
- 1/2 teaspoon vanilla

DIRECTIONS

1. Preheat the oven to 350 f.
2. Line baking dish with parchment paper and set aside.
3. Add all ingredients into the blender and blend until smooth.
4. Pour in the batter into the prepared dish and then bake for 20 minutes.
5. Slice and serve.

Nutritions: Calories 81, Fat 2g, Carbohydrates 10g, Sugar 5.2g, Protein 7g, Cholesterol 15mg

291. GRILLED PEACH SUNDAES

PREPARATION: 5 MIN

COOKING: 0 MIN

SERVES: 1

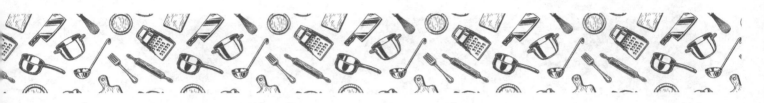

INGREDIENTS

- 1 tablespoon toasted unsweetened coconut
- 1 teaspoon canola oil
- 2 peaches, halved and pitted
- 2 scoops non-fat vanilla yogurt, frozen

DIRECTIONS

1. Brush the peaches with oil and grill until tender.
2. Place peach halves on a bowl and top with frozen yogurt and coconut.

Nutritions: *Calories: 61; Carbs: 2g; Protein: 2g; Fats: 6g; Phosphorus: 32mg; Potassium: 85mg; Sodium: 30mg*

292. BELGIAN WAFFLE WITH FRUITS

PREPARATION: 10 MIN   **COOKING: 25 MIN**   **SERVES: 6**

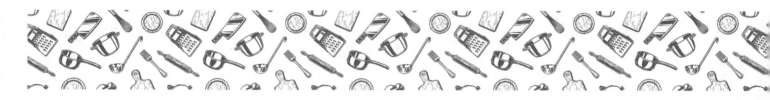

INGREDIENTS

- Eggs – 2 larges
- Cake flour – 2 cups
- Baking soda – ¾ teaspoon
- Sour cream – ¾ cup
- 1% low-fat milk – ¾ cup
- Vanilla extract – 2 teaspoons
- Unsalted butter – 4 tablespoons
- Granulated sugar – 2 tablespoons
- Powdered sugar – 6 tablespoons

DIRECTIONS

1. Start by heating the waffle iron.
2. Now take a large mixing bowl and add in the baking soda and cake flour. Mix well and set aside.
3. Take 2 medium bowls and separate the egg whites and the yolks.
4. Add the vanilla extract and sour cream to the bowl with the egg yolks and whisk well. Add the melted butter and mix well.
5. Take the second bowl with the egg whites. Using a mixer on medium speed, beat the eggs to form soft peaks.
6. Add in the granulated sugar and beat for another 3-4 minutes to form stiff peaks.
7. Whisk together the flour mixture and sour cream mixture to combine well.
8. Add in the egg white mixture and gently fold through.
9. Add approximately ½ cup of batter to the heated waffle iron and close the iron.
10. Cook the mixture for 3 minutes. Once done, empty onto a serving platter.
11. Garnish with powdered sugar, fresh berries, syrup, and whipped cream.

Nutritions: Carbohydrates 50g, Protein 8g, Fat 15g, Sodium 204mg, Cholesterol 98mg, Potassium 151mg Calcium 81mg, Phosphorus 121mg, Fiber 1g

293. PHILLY CHEESE STEAK STUFFED MUSHROOMS

PREPARATION: 15 MIN

COOKING: 15 MIN

SERVES: 2

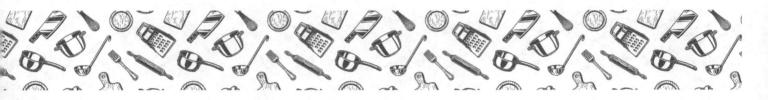

INGREDIENTS

- 24 oz. baby belle mushrooms
- 1 cup chopped red pepper
- 1 cup chopped onion
- 2 tablespoons butter
- 1 teaspoon salt divided
- ½ teaspoon of pepper divided
- 1 pound of beef sirloin shaved or thinly sliced against the grain
- ounces of provolone cheese
- Get Ingredients Powered by Chicory

DIRECTIONS

1. First heat oven to 350 degrees, Remove stems from mushrooms and place mushrooms on a greased baby sheet. Sprinkle with ½ teaspoon of salt and ¼ teaspoon of pepper on both sides and bake for 15 minutes. Set aside.
2. Melt 1 tablespoon butter in a large skillet and cook pepper and onions until soft. Then season with ½ teaspoon of salt and ¼ teaspoon of pepper.
3. Remove from the skillet and set aside. In the same skillet,
4. melt the remaining tablespoon of butter and cook the meat to your preference.
5. Add the provolone cheese and stir until completely melted.
6. Return back the veggies. Add mixture into the mushrooms, top with more cheese if you like and bake for 5 minutes. Serve and enjoy.

Nutritions: *Calories: 435, Fat: 16g, Carbohydrates: 27g, Fiber: 3g, Protein: 39g*

294. SPICY BROCCOLI MACARONI

PREPARATION: 10 MIN

COOKING: 25 MIN

SERVES: 2

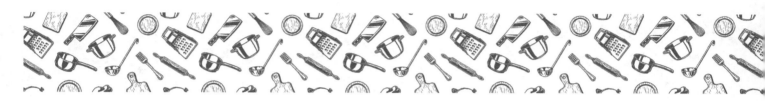

INGREDIENTS

- 1 cup macaroni boiled
- 2 teaspoon garlic, chopped
- 1/2 teaspoon red chilies, chopped
- ¼ cup broccoli
- Pepper
- Olive oil

DIRECTIONS

1. Heat the oil in a pan and sauté the garlic.
2. Add red chilies. Season with salt and pepper.
3. Add broccoli and cook for two minutes.
4. Add boiled macaroni.
5. Cook for 2-3 minutes. Serve hot.

Nutritions: Calories 102, Total Fat 4.6g, Saturated Fat 1.1g, Cholesterol 3mg, Sodium 35mg, Total Carbohydrate 11.9g, Dietary Fiber 0.8g, Total Sugar 0.3g, Protein 3.4g, Calcium 39mg, Iron 0mg, Potassium 39mg, Phosphorus 10 Mg

295. QUICK QUICHE

PREPARATION: 15 MIN

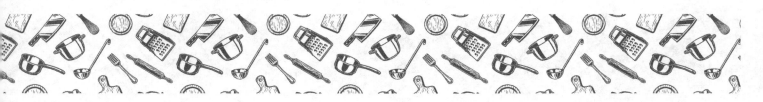

COOKING: 35 MIN

SERVES: 2

INGREDIENTS

- 1 teaspoon olive oil
- 1 egg white, beaten
- 1 tablespoon finely chopped onion
- ¼ teaspoon black pepper
- ¼ cup all-purpose flour
- ½ cup soy milk

DIRECTIONS

1. Preheat oven to 350 degrees f. And then lightly grease a 9-inch pie pan.
2. Combine egg white, olive oil, onion, black pepper, flour and soy milk; whisk together until smooth; pour into pie pan.
3. Bake in preheated oven for 30-35 minutes, until set. Serve hot or cold.

Nutritions: *Calories 121, Total Fat 3.6g, Saturated Fat 0.5g, Cholesterol 0mg, Sodium 48mg, Total Carbohydrate 16.5g, Dietary Fiber 1g, Total Sugar 2.8g, Protein 5.5g, Calcium 21mg, Iron 1mg, Potassium 126mg, Phosphorus 90 Mg*

296. CHOCOLATE TRIFLE

PREPARATION: 20 MIN

COOKING: 15 MIN

SERVES: 4

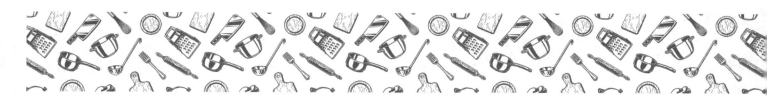

INGREDIENTS

- 1 small plain sponge swiss roll
- oz. Custard powder
- oz. Hot water
- 16 oz. Canned mandarins
- tablespoons sherry
- oz. Double cream
- chocolate squares, grated

DIRECTIONS

1. Whisk the custard powder with water in a bowl until dissolved.
2. In a bowl, mix the custard well until it becomes creamy and let it sit for 15 minutes.
3. Spread the swiss roll and cut it in 4 squares.
4. Place the swiss roll in the 4 serving cups.
5. Top the swiss roll with mandarin, custard, cream, and chocolate.
6. Serve.

Nutritions: Calories 315, Total fat 13.5g, Cholesterol 43mg, Sodium 185mg, Protein 2.9g, Calcium 61mg, Phosphorous 184mg, Potassium 129mg

297. PINEAPPLE MERINGUES

PREPARATION: 10 MIN

COOKING: 0 MIN

SERVES: 4

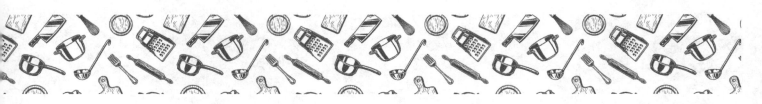

INGREDIENTS

- meringue nests
- oz. Crème fraiche
- 2 oz. Stem ginger, chopped
- oz. Can pineapple chunks

DIRECTIONS

1. Place the meringue nests on the serving plates.
2. Whisk the ginger with crème fraiche and pineapple chunks.
3. Divide this the pineapple mixture over the meringue nests.
4. Serve.

Nutritions: *Calories 312, Cholesterol 0mg, Sodium 41mg, Protein 2.3g, Calcium 3mg, Phosphorous 104mg, Potassium 110mg*

298. BAKED CUSTARD

PREPARATION: 15 MIN

COOKING: 30 MIN

SERVES: 1

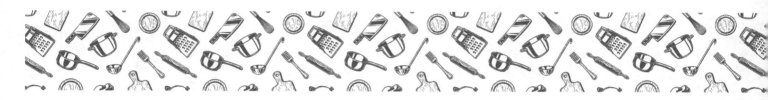

INGREDIENTS

- 1/2 cup milk
- 1 egg, beaten
- 1/8 teaspoon nutmeg
- 1/8 teaspoon vanilla
- Sweetener, to taste
- 1/2 cup water

DIRECTIONS

1. Lightly warm up the milk in a pan, then whisk in the egg, nutmeg, vanilla and sweetener.
2. Pour this custard mixture into a ramekin.
3. Place the ramekin in a baking pan and pour ½ cup water into the pan.
4. Bake the custard for 30 minutes at 325 degrees f.
5. Serve fresh.

Nutritions: Calories 127, Total fat 7g, Cholesterol 174mg, Sodium 119mg, Calcium 169mg, Phosphorous 309mg, Potassium 171mg

299. STRAWBERRY PIE

PREPARATION: 15 MIN

COOKING: 25 MIN

SERVES: 6

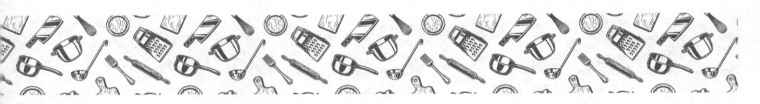

INGREDIENTS

- 1 unbaked (9 inches) pie shell
- cups strawberries, fresh
- 1 cup of brown swerve
- tablespoons arrowroot powder
- 2 tablespoons lemon juice
- tablespoons whipped cream topping

DIRECTIONS

1. Spread the pie shell in the pie pan and bake it until golden brown.
2. Now mash 2 cups of strawberries with the lemon juice, arrowroot powder, and swerve in a bowl.
3. Add the mixture to a saucepan and cook on moderate heat until it thickens.
4. Allow the mixture to cool then spread it in the pie shell.
5. Slice the remaining strawberries and spread them over the pie filling.
6. Refrigerate for 1 hour then garnish with whipped cream.
7. Serve fresh and enjoy.

Nutritions: *Calories 236, Total fat 11.1g, Cholesterol 3mg, Sodium 183mg, Protein 2.2g, Calcium 23mg, Phosphorous 47.2mg, Potassium 178mg*

300. EASY TURNIP PUREE

PREPARATION: 10 MIN

COOKING: 12 MIN

SERVES: 4

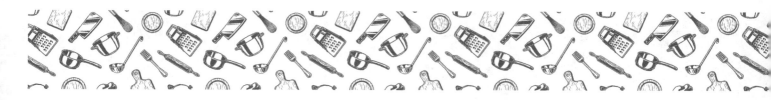

INGREDIENTS

- 1 1/2 lbs. Turnips, peeled and chopped
- 1 tsp dill
- bacon slices, cooked and chopped
- 2 tbsp fresh chives, chopped

DIRECTIONS

1. Add turnip into the boiling water and cook for 12 minutes. Drain well and place in a food processor.
2. Add dill and process until smooth.
3. Transfer turnip puree into the bowl and top with bacon and chives.
4. Serve and enjoy.

Nutritions: calories 127, fat 6g, carbohydrates 11.6g, sugar 7g, protein 6.8g, cholesterol 16mg

301. SPINACH BACON BAKE

PREPARATION: 10 MIN

COOKING: 45 MIN

SERVES: 6

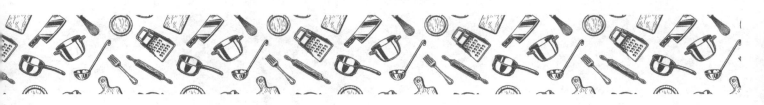

INGREDIENTS

- eggs
- cups baby spinach, chopped
- 1 tbsp olive oil
- bacon slices, cooked and chopped
- 2 tomatoes, sliced
- 2 tbsp chives, chopped
- Pepper
- Salt

DIRECTIONS

1. Preheat the oven to 350 f.
2. Spray a baking dish with cooking spray and set aside.
3. Heat oil in a pan.
4. Add spinach and cook until spinach wilted.
5. In a mixing bowl, whisk eggs and salt. Add spinach and chives and stir well.
6. Pour egg mixture into the baking dish.
7. Top with tomatoes and bacon and bake for 45 minutes.
8. Serve and enjoy.

Nutritions: *Calories 273, Fat 20.4g, Carbohydrates 3.1g, Sugar 1.7g, Protein 19.4g, Cholesterol 301mg*

302. HEALTHY SPINACH TOMATO MUFFINS

PREPARATION: 10 MIN

COOKING: 20 MIN

SERVES: 12

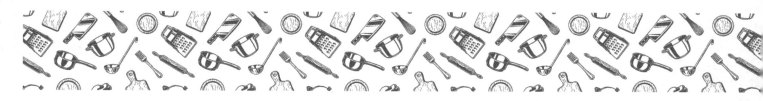

INGREDIENTS

- eggs
- 1/2 tsp italian seasoning
- 1 cup tomatoes, chopped
- tbsp water
- 1 cup fresh spinach, chopped
- Pepper
- Salt

DIRECTIONS

1. Preheat the oven to 350 f.
2. Spray muffin tray with cooking spray and set aside.
3. In a mixing bowl, whisk eggs with water, italian seasoning, pepper, and salt.
4. Add spinach and tomatoes and stir well.
5. Pour egg mixture into the prepared muffin tray and bake for 20 minutes.
6. Serve and enjoy.

Nutritions: Calories 67, Fat 4.5g, Carbohydrates 1g, Sugar 0.8g, Protein 5.7g, Cholesterol 164mg

CHAPTER 15.
MEA SUREMENTS AND CONVERSION

Volume

Imperial	Metric	Imperial	Metric
1 tbsp	15ml	1 pint	570 ml
2 fl oz	55 ml	1 ¼ pints	725 ml
3 fl oz	75 ml	1 ¾ pints	1 liter
5 fl oz (¼ pint)	150 ml	2 pints	1.2 liters
10 fl oz (½ pint)	275 ml	2½ pints	1.5 liters
		4 pints	2.25 liters

Weight

Imperial	Metric	Imperial	Metric	Imperial	Metric
½ oz	10 g	4 oz	110 g	10 oz	275 g
¾ oz	20 g	4½ oz	125 g	12 oz	350 g
1 oz	25 g	5 oz	150 g	1 lb	450 g
1½ oz	40 g	6 oz	175 g	1 lb 8 oz	700 g
2 oz	50 g	7 oz	200 g	2 lb	900 g
2½ oz	60 g	8 oz	225 g	3 lb	1.35 kg
3 oz	75 g	9 oz	250 g		

Metric cups conversion

Cups	Imperial	Metric
1 cup flour	5oz	150g
1 cup caster or granulated sugar	8oz	225g
1 cup soft brown sugar	6oz	175g
1 cup soft butter/margarine	8oz	225g
1 cup sultanas/raisins	7oz	200g
1 cup currants	5oz	150g
1 cup ground almonds	4oz	110g
1 cup oats	4oz	110g
1 cup golden syrup/honey	12oz	350g
1 cup uncooked rice	7oz	200g
1 cup grated cheese	4oz	110g
1 stick butter	4oz	110g
¼ cup liquid (water, milk, oil etc.)	4 tablespoons	60ml
½ cup liquid (water, milk, oil etc.)	¼ pint	125ml
1 cup liquid (water, milk, oil etc.)	½ pint	250ml

Oven temperatures

Gas Mark	Fahrenheit	Celsius	Gas Mark	Fahrenheit	Celsius
1/4	225	110	4	350	180
1/2	250	130	5	375	190
1	275	140	6	400	200
2	300	150	7	425	220
3	325	170	8	450	230
			9	475	240

Weight

Imperial	Metric	Imperial	Metric
½ oz	10 g	6 oz	175 g
¾ oz	20 g	7 oz	200 g
1 oz	25 g	8 oz	225 g
1½ oz	40 g	9 oz	250 g
2 oz	50 g	10 oz	275 g
2½ oz	60 g	12 oz	350 g
3 oz	75 g	1 lb	450 g
4 oz	110 g	1 lb 8 oz	700 g
4½ oz	125 g	2 lb	900 g
5 oz	150 g	3 lb	1.35 kg

CONCLUSION

You likely had little knowledge about your kidneys before. You probably didn't know how you could take steps to improve your kidney health and decrease the risk of developing kidney failure. However, you now understand the power of the human kidney, as well as the prognosis of chronic kidney disease. While over thirty-million Americans are being affected by kidney disease, you can now take steps to be one of the people who are actively working to promote your kidney health. Kidney disease now ranks as the 18th deadliest condition in the world. In the United States alone, it is reported that over 600,000 Americans succumb to kidney failure.

These stats are alarming, which is why, it is necessary to take proper care of your kidneys, starting with a kidney-friendly diet. These recipes are ideal whether you have been diagnosed with a kidney problem or you want to prevent any kidney issue.

As for your well-being and health, it's a good idea to see your doctor as often as possible to make sure you don't have any preventable problems you don't need to have. The kidneys are your body's channel for toxins (as is the liver), cleaning the blood of unknown substances and toxins that are removed from things like preservatives in the food and other toxins. The moment you eat without control and fill your body with toxins, food, drink (liquor or alcohol, for example) or even the air you inhale in general, your body will also convert a number of things that appear to be benign until the body's organs convert them to things like formaldehyde, due to a synthetic response and transformation phase.

One such case is a large part of the dietary sugars used in diet sodas - for example, aspartame is converted to formaldehyde in the body. These toxins must be excreted or they can cause disease, renal (kidney) failure, malignant growth, and various other painful problems

This isn't a condition that occurs without any forethought it is a dynamic issue and in that it very well may be both found early and treated, diet changed, and settling what is causing the issue is conceivable. It's conceivable to have partial renal failure yet, as a rule; it requires some time (or downright poor diet for a short time) to arrive at absolute renal failure. You would prefer not to reach total renal failure since this will require standard dialysis treatments to save your life.

Dialysis treatments explicitly clean the blood of waste and toxins in the blood utilizing a machine in light of the fact that your body can no longer carry out the responsibility. Without treatments, you could die a very painful death. Renal failure can be the consequence of long-haul diabetes, hypertension, unreliable diet, and can stem from other health concerns.

A renal diet is tied in with directing the intake of protein and phosphorus in your eating routine. Restricting your sodium intake is likewise significant. By controlling these two variables you can control the vast majority of the toxins/waste made by your body and thus this enables your kidney to 100% function. In the event that you get this early enough and truly moderate your diets with extraordinary consideration, you could avert complete renal failure. In the event that you get this early, you can take out the issue completely.

CPSIA information can be obtained
at www.ICGtesting.com
Printed in the USA
LVHW022242181220
674519LV00011B/540